Praise for *The End of Overeating*

"A fascinating account of the science of human appetite, as well as its exploitation by the food industry. *The End of Overeating* is an invaluable contribution to the national conversation about the catastrophe that is the modern American diet."
—Michael Pollan, author of *In Defense of Food*

"David Kessler's bestseller, *The End of Overeating*, is both a thinking person's diet book and an investigation into an industry that wants us to eat more."
—*Boston Globe*

"Fascinating. . . . Dr. Kessler offers practical advice for using the science of overeating to our advantage, so that we begin to think about food and take back control of our eating habits."
—*The New York Times*

"Disturbing, thought-provoking, and important."
—Anthony Bourdain

"In perversely fascinating detail, Kessler . . . reveals how industrial chefs engineered . . . 'hyperpalatable' concoctions undreamed of in any traditional cuisine."
—*The New York Times Book Review*

"Fascinating exploration of us . . . we begin to think differently about food and take back control of our eating habits."
—Tara Parker-Pope, *The New York Times*

"In a wide-ranging look at eating habits, David Kessler, the former head of the Food and Drug Administration, addresses America's ever-increasing waistlines."
—*The Wall Street Journal*

"Groundbreaking."
—*USA Today*

FOOD OR FICTION?

ALSO BY DAVID A. KESSLER, MD

Capture

The End of Overeating

A Question of Intent

FOOD OR FICTION?

The Truth About the Ultraprocessed
Foods Making America Sick

David A. Kessler, MD

HARPER

NEW YORK • LONDON • TORONTO • SYDNEY

HARPER

FIRST HARPER PAPERBACKS EDITION PUBLISHED 2024.

The Library of Congress has catalogued the hardcover edition as follows:

Names: Kessler, David A., author.

Title: Fast carbs, slow carbs: the simple truth about food, weight, and disease / David A. Kessler.

Description: First edition. | New York : HarperWave, [2020] | Includes bibliographical references and index. | Summary: "The American body is plagued by obesity, heart disease, and diabetes. In Fast Carbs, Slow Carbs, the follow up to his bestselling book The End of Overeating, Dr. David A. Kessler explains how we can reduce heart disease, keep weight off, and reduce chronic disease"—Provided by publisher.

Identifiers: LCCN 2019052571 (print) | LCCN 2019052572 (ebook) | ISBN 9780062996978 (hardback) | ISBN 9780062996992 (ebook)

Subjects: LCSH: Carbohydrates in human nutrition—Popular works. | Carbohydrates, Refined—Physiological effect. | Processed foods—United States—Popular works. | Nutritionally induced diseases—United States–Popular works.

Classification: LCC TX553.C28 K47 2020 (print) | LCC TX553.C28 (ebook) | DDC 615.8/54—dc23

LC record available at https://lccn.loc.gov/2019052571 LC ebook record available at https://lccn.loc.gov/2019052572

978-0-06-338257-2 (pbk.)

24 25 26 27 28 LBC 5 4 3 2 1

For Lena and David

Contents

Part IV Metabolic Chaos

Part V Heart Disease

Preface

As this book was first being published in 2020, the United States declared a public health emergency due to the SARS-CoV-2 virus. I was enlisted to help with the national response, and on January 20, 2021, I joined the White House COVID-19 response team and helped lead Operation Warp Speed, which was responsible for the nation's vaccine and antiviral drug effort. I was, as were we all, confronted with two epidemics: one, new, from an infectious virus; the other, of decades' duration, from chronic diseases, including heart disease, diabetes, and cancer, that result from excess body weight. As I would learn, the two epidemics were linked, with individuals with excess weight being more vulnerable to the devastating effects of COVID-19. While the death rate from COVID-19 has come down as we've gained immunity as the result of both vaccines and natural immunity, we have not made any progress with weight-related chronic diseases. The Center for Disease Control has announced that obesity remains on the rise in a growing number of states, with twenty-two states having an obesity rate of 35 percent or more.

The food we eat and the weight we gain from that food cause nearly five hundred thousand annual deaths in the Unted States. More than a decade ago, I wrote *The End of Overeating*, which focused on the role of highly palatable foods and how the food industry designs those foods to keep us eating. In this book, I concentrate on highly processed foods and how the food industry uses processing to make food highly palatable and energy dense, with more calories packed into the food. Together, highly processed, highly palatable foods that are energy dense are the cause of the obesity epidemic.

New research during the last several years continues to support this book's thesis that these foods throw our body into metabolic chaos. We have known, through the work of Dr. Kevin Hall at the National Institutes of Health, that people eat about five hundred more calories per day and gain more weight when consuming ultraprocessed food. What is new is the finding that both hyper-palatability and energy density, just as we predicted, are associated with that increased intake. Also supported, as we discuss in this book, is the importance of a food's structure. New research shows that "fast" foods that have less structure and can be eaten more quickly contribute 22% more calories to our diets than "slow" foods that are consumed less rapidly. Food processing generally affects the structure of food and increases caloric intake.

We were able to get the COVID-19 epidemic under control. We have long needed a call to action to tackle the epidemic of chronic disease caused by the processed food we eat. That action can only be spurred by an accepted understanding of what lies at the root of the problem. As this book shows, most of the damage caused by highly processed, highly palatable food is driven by "fast" carbs, but the problem is not just carbohydrates. Processed foods that are high in combinations of fat and salt, fat and sugar, and carbs and salt are also major drivers of increased caloric intake. In recent decades, the composition of many food items has been changed to increase palatability, resulting in a marked increase in the availability of hyperpalatable foods. These foods are prevalent in our food supply, now making up almost 60 percent of the US food system, and an estimated 67 percent of the total energy intake in children and adolescents aged two through nineteen. It is why evidence of metabolic and cardiovascular disease is showing up earlier in life.

What we call "food" is, in large part, no longer simply what sustains us and what we enjoy. Its fundamental nature has changed and it is killing us. How we have looked at this catastrophic takeover of what we eat, which has such an enormous impact on our health, begs the question: Is what we eat food or fiction? Thus, the new title of this book.

Introduction:
The Birth of Fast Carbs

Grain is an American archetype, a symbol of the United States as a breadbasket to the world. Its influence in our history and economic development can scarcely be exaggerated.

A stucco frieze on the ceiling of the New Room at Mount Vernon, the mansion owned by George Washington, showcases a sheaf of wheat. In a letter to Lafayette on June 18, 1788, Washington wrote, "I hope, some day or another we shall become a storehouse and granary for the world." Abraham Lincoln created the U.S. Department of Agriculture and established land grant colleges to promote agricultural education. Since 1887, when Congress passed the Hatch Act, professionals assigned to every farming county in the nation have been charged with ensuring that the nation's farmers have the assets they need to extract the largest return possible from the land, with the greatest efficiency.

In short, the federal government has played a central role in shaping American agriculture since the nation's birth. As a result, we have built a vast economic infrastructure on starch. It began with the westward expansion in the nineteenth century and accelerated rapidly in the twentieth, taking full advantage of fertile prairie grasslands and of other conditions that enabled wheat and corn cultivation to thrive in the fields of the Midwest and West.

Decades before refrigeration, the continental railroad system seemed purpose-built for shipping sacks of uniform, easily traded grain. The tractor and mechanized farm equipment made possible the near-automation of grain harvesting; fruit and vegetable production, by contrast, still mostly depends on human labor.

After World War II, the large-scale explosives factories that could use the air's nitrogen to make ammonia were reconfigured to manufacture commercial fertilizer, which could be spread on the vast grasslands. And in his bid for reelection in 1972, Richard Nixon transformed the federal farm subsidy program, giving American farmers an incentive to grow as much starch as they possibly could.

Consumer culture grew in parallel to industrial agriculture. Food companies found they could make considerable profits by selling processed foods. Then they stumbled upon the Holy Grail of food engineering, discovering ways to make food irresistible to the majority of Americans. With the right combinations of starch, fat, sugar, and salt, they could get people to keep eating—and purchasing—their products. They had a willing partner in the starch production industry, which excelled at processing whole grains into fast carbs.

The expanding starch marketing apparatus received one more boon from the federal government in the form of well-intentioned dietary guidelines that unwittingly directed Americans to eat more highly processed starch.

Although direct payments to farmers have ended, American farm policy helped spawn a starch production and marketing behemoth that dominated the food landscape, as it continues to do today. Large corporations and conglomerates now control every step of the food chain, from the fields to the processing plants to the fast food establishments that sell us supersize, starch-based meals. That is the inescapable food environment in which we live, the sea of starch in which we struggle to stay healthy.

Yet we can also detect strong signs of positive change in our culture. Consumer demand for organic produce, organic food, and products without added sugar continues to rise. The twin epidemics of obesity and diabetes are fixed in the public consciousness. Growing numbers of Americans now stand in the aisles of their supermarkets, as I have done, studying food labels. With billions of dollars at stake, much of the food processing industry has responded with, unsurprisingly, more processed food. They have slapped "clean" and "natural" labels on their products and replaced chemically modified starches with naturally occurring or physically altered starches with names that don't broadcast their chemical contents. They've created low-glycemic processed foods, plant-based processed foods, and processed foods with added fiber, tinkering and reformulating around the edges without abandoning their dependence on processed starch. But none of that addresses the core problem of fast carbs.

Part I

Trapped in Food Chaos

Chapter 1

———

An extraordinary
opportunity to save lives

The fields of wheat and rows of corn and soy that quilt the American heartland are a source of national pride and a feat of ingenuity and technology. We can grow enough food for the entire country and beyond, and employ hundreds of thousands of people to cultivate, process, and package it until it arrives at our supermarkets. This system allows each of us to live without having to forage for sustenance, plant our own gardens, keep our own livestock, or worry about how to feed ourselves when winter comes.

The earth, of course, is the source of this bounty. It offers itself up to us in the form of grain, fruits, and vegetables. That it produces the exact nutrients our bodies need to thrive is the unfathomable result of evolution. If we imagine the earth as a living, cognizant entity, we might think that it wants us to survive. That it cares about us. *Why* this is may always be a mystery, but we are in a deep and inextricable relationship with the earth, one in which we humans should be flourishing.

Yet despite the healthy sustenance available to us, we are far from healthy. Americans are plagued by obesity, heart disease, and diabetes, and incredibly, our food has become the number one cause of these ailments. Not food in its natural, unprocessed state, but the products that emerge from the huge processing plants that also dot the heartland. The food processing industry has destroyed the inherent structure of food, transforming much of it into highly palatable, ultraprocessed carbohydrates that can be digested rapidly. We, in turn, are consuming these rapidly digestible carbs—starches and sugar, which I refer to as *fast carbs*—in larger and larger quantities, and they are destroying our bodies. Globally, eleven million deaths and 250 million disabilities are attributable to diet; that translates into one in five deaths.

In the pages ahead, I'll build the case for the many kinds of damage that result from consuming these foods, but the capsule view is this: fast carbs hijack appetite, interfere with feelings of fullness, make it hard to control weight, and have a toxic effect on metabolic pathways, which results in a vicious cycle of insulin resistance, obesity, and chronic disease. The American diet also increases our odds of developing heart disease.

While human biology is complex, the road to better health doesn't have to be. The goal of this book is to cut through the confusion surrounding food, diet, and health. Identifying the danger posed by fast carbs will allow us to reclaim a healthy body weight, prevent diabetes, and markedly reduce atherosclerotic heart disease. The information here is aimed at people who, like me, have engaged in a lifelong struggle with weight, but it will also be useful to anyone who is interested in eating a healthy diet.

It's important to understand that ultraprocessed foods are designed to be irresistible, and to prompt overconsumption. In addition to degrading the structure of carbohydrates, food processors increase the palatability, or sensory appeal, of these already compromised foods by adding sugar, fat, and salt. Virtually all packaged snack foods feature some combination of those ingredients, as do pizza, fries, and many baked products. Once we start eating them, it's very difficult to stop; that's because we absorb fast carbs early and quickly in our gastrointestinal tracts. As a result, our bodies don't release the hormones that trigger fullness—and we keep on eating. It's a vicious cycle.

But overeating isn't the only health hazard posed by fast carbs. They also elevate blood glucose levels, which then cause insulin levels to rise. That leads to increasing dysfunction of the metabolic pathways, which are the linked chemical reactions that occur in the body, including how we process the foods we eat and the reactions that convert them into the energy and molecules we need to live.

By continuing to eat fast carbs, we further accelerate this dysfunction. Eventually, the body becomes less sensitive to the presence of insulin, which is essential to controlling blood glucose. This can lead to metabolic syndrome, insulin resistance, prediabetes, and ultimately a diagnosis of full-blown type 2 diabetes. The package of consequences that can occur when normal metabolism is disrupted is referred to as metabolic disease.

A related threat to our bodies is caused by blood lipids, especially low-density lipoproteins (LDL), which are toxic particles that are the leading cause of cardiovascular disease. The importance of understanding this is twofold. First, when you limit your intake of fast carbs, it is important not to replace them with saturated fat, which can increase LDL in our blood. Second, research tells us that lowering LDL levels offers us a life-altering opportunity to prevent cardiovascular disease.

There are three major recommendations in this book. They are more direct than any national dietary guidelines, and they are strongly supported by the latest science. Embrace these recommendations for the long term and you'll achieve lasting change in your weight and your health. Study after study has shown that if you lose excess weight and keep it off, you can reverse diabetes and other diseases that occur when normal metabolism is disrupted, and prevent cardiovascular disease.

Here are the three recommendations:

1. **Reduce consumption of fast carbs to gain control over weight and reduce the risk of metabolic disease.**

2. **Reduce your blood lipids (especially LDL) by moving to a largely plant-based diet or by taking**

medications to markedly diminish the risk of
cardiovascular disease.

3. Engage in daily moderate-intensity exercise to
control weight, increase metabolic flexibility, and
reduce the risk of metabolic and cardiovascular
disease.

That's it. Simple and direct. But these recommendations
emerge from a systematic, in-depth investigation that took
me years to complete. During that time, I interviewed
dozens of experts, attended conferences around the world,
and reviewed a vast body of medical literature. I especially
relied, where possible, on randomized controlled trials,
which represent the most rigorous scientific method available for comparing diets.

Armed with an understanding of the dangers posed by
fast carbs, and the knowledge of what you can do to avoid
them, I believe we can finally break the cycle of weight loss
and gain that torments so many of us. We can take control
of our bodies and start on a path toward health, greatly
reducing the dangers posed by obesity, diabetes, and heart
disease and restoring sanity to our diets. Not since the
public health campaigns against tobacco have we had such
an extraordinary opportunity to save lives.

Chapter 2

———

There is a path out of the lifelong trap of food chaos that leads to lasting weight loss and health

I'm a doctor with a lifetime of experience in the field of nutrition and health, but for most of my life I have been trapped in a body that I could neither control nor understand. Food has been my nemesis. Overeating has been my curse. As much as I've studied and learned about the body and about the mechanisms of weight loss, it took decades before I began to feel in control of my own weight. Even now, I sometimes struggle.

I can't remember how old I was when my overeating began. But I know for a long time I ate to feel better, to ease discomfort, and to calm anxiety. I ate for reasons I can't even identify. And when I did, it left me in a state of zoned-out bliss. I could finally relax. Of course, that bliss never lasted long. I came back to reality, crumbs on my shirt, thinking about my next meal, or snack, or piece of candy.

When the urge to eat grew, self-control escaped me. Time was suspended. All that existed was the pizza or burger in front of me, or the chocolate cake I knew would come next. I didn't care if there were consequences to my actions if that pizza was what I truly wanted. I was in thrall to it, plain and simple, and I was going to eat.

This lack of control filled me with regret. For a long time, I was disgusted with myself for not having the willpower to control my behavior around food. It was as if a switch went on in my brain that triggered my eating, and I couldn't turn it off.

I fought with myself to stay on diets, to curb my urges, and sometimes I did manage to lose weight. Sometimes, I even lost a lot of weight. When that happened, I felt transformed, as if being able to reach the last hole on my belt held some deep significance. But usually, my weight loss lasted only for six months or so. Within a year, I would gain it back, and the disgust would return. Over and over again, I would ask myself, *How did I let this happen?* I'd stare at my heavy frame in the mirror and feel the tightness of a shirt or pair of pants that used to fit. I'd despair that all my efforts to lose the weight had been wasted and now I was back to where I started, or perhaps even heavier than before.

I know I am not alone. For those of us struggling with our weight, modern life is an obstacle course—one in which we are expected to jump over the sea of fries and muffins to find our way to a head of lettuce lying limply in the surf. More than two-thirds of Americans are either overweight or obese, and the odds are stacked against us as we face the onslaught of a multibillion-dollar processed food marketing machine.

The medical community has offered little help. It's absurd that despite the fact that obesity is on the rise around the world, the best advice doctors and nutritionists have to offer is still "eat less, exercise more." The sad truth is that many medical experts believe that the body has self-regulating systems that make it virtually impossible to lose weight and keep it off. They may not say so publicly, but that assumption has posed huge barriers to action. As I left one talk on nutrition at a medical conference, I asked the physician lecturer why he hadn't spent more time discussing obesity treatments. His response: trying to treat that is a fool's errand. Despite my own challenges, I still refused to believe he was right.

I desperately needed to figure out how to break down these kinds of barriers and fix my own issues with weight. I was determined to discover the key to waking up in the morning without thinking about food, to shut off the countless messages pushing me to eat. All I wanted was to sit down to breakfast, lunch, and dinner in a sensible and routine way, and perhaps even find lasting sustenance in my meals. I wanted to find a way out of the food chaos that was consuming me.

That was how I felt for decades. The book I wrote on the subject, *The End of Overeating*, offered scientific proof that overeating is caused not by a lack of willpower, but rather by the reward system in our brains that is triggered by cues in the environment, such as smells, sights, or location. In the course of that research, I learned that the multibillion-dollar processed food industry has discovered how to engineer foods to trigger an endless eating loop—in other words, foods designed to make us overeat. The biology of this reward network, and the ways in which it is triggered by certain foods, is now well established.

Understanding the science that is involved in overeating helped me better understand my own behavior. Those cues had interacted with my brain chemistry to capture my attention and set off insatiable urges to eat. Seeking the resulting reward again and again, I mindlessly ate cookie after cookie. The neural circuitry involved in this response is the same one that dictates our physiological response to sex, drugs, and gambling. The ongoing debate in my head—*Should I eat this? Maybe not . . . or just a bit*—stems from cross talk between the rational, logical part of my brain and this powerful reward network that is at the core of our emotional brain.

Yet despite all I had learned, I still found myself caught in the same vicious cycle. I lost weight only to gain it back. But I didn't give up. I knew there had to be a way to make a lasting change. So I set out once again to find a path that led me out of food chaos. I was determined to find the missing piece of the puzzle, though no one seemed to know where it was. Not doctors, not dietitians, not the experts who had designed the national dietary guidelines.

The answer, as it turned out, was right in front of me. After all, when I served as the commissioner of the U.S.

Food and Drug Administration (FDA), I had helped design the Nutrition Facts label that appears today on all packaged foods. That label was part of our attempt to educate consumers, to make them aware of what was in their food so that they could make better choices. But what we had missed in designing that label was the danger lurking in the most common ingredient in our food—highly processed and highly absorbable carbohydrates, or fast carbs.

Chapter 3

———

Until we learn the truth about fast carbs, we won't break the weight loss-and-gain cycle

For decades, people like me were told that the problem of weight gain was just one of arithmetic. If you eat more calories than you burn, you will add pounds. But the science of eating, hunger, and obesity turns out to be much more complicated than that.

One of the most significant scientific discoveries in the past decade is the knowledge that our digestive tract doesn't merely function as an engine that burns fuel. It is a complex hormonal system that handles different types of foods differently, a remarkable sensory organ with its own network of nerve cells, and home to colonies of micro-organisms that help digestion in ways we are still discovering. All of this new information has slowly begun to change our views of diet and health as we realize that *what* we eat matters almost as much as the *amount* we eat.

Now, when I stand in the supermarket with a box of breakfast cereal in my hand and look at the ingredients, I realize that the label does not really describe what is in the box. It may say "whole grain," but often that is not true. The grain in that cereal, and in so many other packages, has been highly processed. It's likely been broken up into component parts and reassembled. Most important, its biological structure has been changed. The label explains none of this.

Of course, humans have been processing food for hundreds of thousands of years. Every time you cook something, you are "processing" it, changing its chemical structure to make it easier to chew, digest, and absorb. But in the modern industrial food chain, food is being processed in ways that we have never seen before. Rather than simply grinding grain into smaller pieces to produce flour, manufacturers often subject the grain to intense heat and milling in a series of steps that change the structure of the carbohydrate molecules. These highly processed carbohydrates are essentially predigested when they arrive in the supermarket. As we eat them, our digestive system is flooded with glucose molecules—sugar—that are rapidly absorbed by the body.

Like so many people who struggle with weight, I have been consuming far more of these fast carbs than my body can tolerate. Predigested starches are everywhere in the food system, and they are the primary source of calories in many of our diets. This endless stream of quickly absorbed glucose wreaks havoc on the digestive and hormonal systems, affecting not only our weight but also our risk of developing diabetes and cardiovascular disease. The facts about fast carbs, and the way they have come to dominate our diet, are the missing information we need to break the cycle of weight loss and gain and achieve lasting health.

Chapter 4

———

The problem posed by
highly processed (fast) carbs has
been suspected for decades

My "discovery" about the health problems posed by fast carbs is not really a discovery at all. The arguments against eating refined grains, and rapidly absorbable carbohydrates, date back to the mid-nineteenth century. In 1837, the preacher and temperance leader Sylvester Graham cautioned his followers to avoid white flour, advising them to only eat bread made with the whole grain flour that celebrated the goodness of nature.

Over a century later, the debate about white flour was still raging. In the 1960s, it was taken up by Overeaters Anonymous (OA), a twelve-step program for compulsive eaters. The leaders of OA recognized the same cycle of overeating that I and so many others have experienced. In their view, obesity was caused by intense, irresistible cravings that dissipated only with a "hit" of food. The relief was always temporary, and then the urge came back with ferocious intensity. People who suffered from the disorder of overeating ate mindlessly, endlessly, entering a realm in which, if only for a moment, they no longer cared about their behavior. But of course, they felt worse after such a binge: embarrassed by lack of control, overcome by shame and disgust.

Overeaters Anonymous was founded by Rozanne S., who attended a Gamblers Anonymous meeting in 1958. Listening to the compulsive gamblers share their struggles, she recognized the same cycle she was experiencing as an overeater. The problem was that while the gambler could abstain from gambling and still live, a human could not forgo all food and expect to survive. Rozanne soon began to host OA meetings.

Meanwhile, Father Edward Dowling, a Jesuit priest who served as sponsor and spiritual adviser to Bill Wilson, the cofounder of Alcoholics Anonymous, described a similar moment of reckoning. "My 240-pound gluttony gave me two heart attacks," he wrote. "A doctor who was also a recovering alcoholic got me down toward 180 pounds when he advised the total abstinence from starch, butter, salt, and sugar. He said these four foods were probably my alcohol." Two of the foods on that list—starch and sugar—are fast carbs.

After reading Father Dowling's writings, one of the original members of OA drew the same connection. "I feel I have an allergy to carbohydrates, just as the alcoholic is allergic to alcohol," she wrote. It was an instinctive idea that did not yet have any foundation in clinical studies. Even so, she found that abstaining from carbs made her less preoccupied with them, and she went on to lose seventy pounds.

Many members of OA stumbled onto an effective method for avoiding processed carbs—they "crunched all day on low-calorie foods," often obsessively, said one member. They nibbled on carrots or celery, in effect substituting intact, unprocessed vegetables for predigested fast carbs. For decades, leaders of the organization debated about whether to recommend abstinence from processed carbohydrates as a part of the program. They circulated a plan to do so, but ultimately concluded that such a recommendation lacked any scientific basis and abandoned it.

In the time since then, much research has been published on diet and nutrition. And yet at any gathering at which these topics are discussed, including conferences of eminent scientists, you will still hear fierce debates about what constitutes the optimal diet. The search for a consensus has, to date, eluded us. Meanwhile, generations of Americans continue to eat fast carbs in great quantities and continue to suffer the effects of ill health.

Chapter 5

———

Only 12.2 percent of Americans
are metabolically healthy

A few dozen people were with me at a Nashville, Tennessee, conference when Dr. Joana Araujo presented her analysis of National Health and Nutrition Examination Survey data between 2009 and 2016. But what Dr. Araujo, a young postdoctoral research associate in nutrition from the University of North Carolina at Chapel Hill, told us deserves a place in headlines across the country. She revealed a shocking statistic: only 12.2 percent of Americans are metabolically healthy. That means seven out of every eight of us are at significant risk for developing major diseases, including diabetes and cardiovascular disease.

I wish there had been thousands of clinicians and public health professionals in the room to hear that stunning finding. A worldwide epidemic of disease is unfolding, and it is largely the result of what we are eating. Food-related illnesses aren't limited to diabetes and heart disease; they also include health concerns such as blood clots, low testosterone, erectile dysfunction, inflammation, infertility, irregular menses, gout, gallstones, acne, fatty liver disease, and stroke.

These ailments involve different biological mechanisms but they are all rooted in the same problem: excess body fat. Dr. Harold Bays, who studies both cardiovascular and metabolic disease, explains it this way: "When you increase body fat, your fat cells get sick. You get sick fat." This causes damage in muscle and in the liver and finally leads to pathological responses. In other words, excess body fat does more than give you extra weight to carry around, putting strain on your heart and joints. Fat cells produce compounds that lead to all sorts of metabolic illness and damage other tissues. When fat cells become sick, they release more fatty acids and other molecules into the blood, creating a ripple effect that disrupts normal body chemical reactions.

This is why ending obesity is not a matter of vanity; it's a matter of life or death. I would like nothing more than to reassure people that they can achieve good health at any size. But regrettably, the scientific evidence just doesn't support this concept, especially as we age. Excess weight is the primary driver for type 2 diabetes and an independent risk factor for heart disease, including heart failure, coronary disease, stroke, and atrial fibrillation—separate and apart from the risk added by high blood pressure and diabetes. Even if you are physically fit, excess weight adds additional risk. It takes about fifteen years for the increased risk to manifest itself. After twenty-five to thirty years of carrying the excess weight, the risk becomes significant. Even if you're not obese but merely overweight, losing excess body fat is the most important thing you can do for your health.

Part II

How Food Stopped
Sustaining Us

Over the past half century, Americans have greatly increased their average daily intake of processed carbohydrates

The twin epidemics of obesity and chronic disease are relatively recent phenomena. For most of human history, adult weight varied little over much of a lifetime. That's because, *given a diet comprising naturally occurring foods*, our bodies' hormonal systems keep us at a healthy weight.

But everything changes when we eat processed foods that are completely foreign to what we have evolved to digest. That is a profound realization, and one that should alter our perspective: we eat for sustenance, but what we consume does not sustain us. According to colleagues at the Centers for Disease Control and Prevention (CDC), the shift began in the 1970s, when the average weight of Americans started to rise steadily. By the early 2000s, many of us were entering our twenties about twenty pounds heavier than people had been just a few decades earlier, and that trend continues today. Rather than stabilizing as we grow into adulthood, we keep gaining weight as we get older. That generally continues until we move into old age, when we tend to shed pounds.

This marked shift lines up with two notable changes in our diet. According to the best data the Department of Agriculture has, in 1970, Americans were availing themselves of 430 calories a day of flour, rice, and cereal products; by 2008, that figure had jumped to 641 calories. At the same time, per capita daily consumption of fats and oils rose from 346 calories in 1970 to 575 calories in 2010. Meanwhile, other food sources stayed relatively constant. For example, the calories from added sugars or sweeteners remained almost unchanged (sugars increased through 1999 and then decreased), though more of them came from corn sweeteners, including high-fructose corn syrup. Also unchanged has been the amount of red meat, poultry, fish, and dairy we eat, as well as our consumption of vegetables and fruit. Only calories from fast carbs and fats have increased.

Today, ultraprocessed foods containing fast carbs and fats constitute about 60 percent of the average daily energy intake of Americans, and sales of these products grow every year. Fast carbs constitute more than 40 percent of our energy intake. Dr. Susan Tosh, professor of food science at the University of Ottawa, sums it up this way: "My thought is that, over the past fifteen to twenty years, we're eating a lot more hamburger buns and sandwiches and French fries and pizza. In other words, the amount of processed carbohydrates has increased in our diet."

Dr. Julie Jones is professor of nutrition at Saint Catherine University and an expert on dietary fiber and starches. "I call them doodles, ding dongs, and donuts," she said. "That is the problem . . . the indulgent grains."

When she speaks of "indulgent grains," Dr. Jones is referring to fast carbs. To understand how they came to occupy such a large part of our diet, we need to take a look back over the past fifty years. Ironically, part of the explanation lies in well-meaning attempts to make us healthier.

Chapter 7

A turning point for our diet

Until the 1970s, discussion of nutrition in America—if there was any discussion at all—was focused on *malnutrition*, a condition caused by not getting adequate food or micronutrients. In 1964, President Lyndon Johnson announced a "War on Poverty" as part of his Great Society program. New policy commitments followed alarming reports in the press about hunger-related diseases in the U.S., including a CBS documentary entitled *Hunger in America*, which shocked many Americans with its depiction of utter deprivation.

In the wake of these reports, U.S. senators George McGovern, Ted Kennedy, and Hubert Humphrey sought to improve the state of nutrition in America. Along with several colleagues, these men made up the Senate Select Committee on Nutrition and Human Needs, also known as the McGovern Committee, named for its chair. From 1968 to 1977, they embarked on a project that was both controversial and revolutionary. For the first time, they established dietary goals designed to influence the eating habits of all Americans.

The initial goal of the McGovern Committee was to fight hunger and malnutrition. Among other laudable efforts, it pushed to expand the reach of food stamps and to establish the federal school lunch program. But by 1973 its attention had broadened to include what was then a relatively new idea—that some Americans were consuming *too much* rather than too little. This coincided with emerging scientific research about the links between diet and heart disease, which captured the committee's interest.

They had good reason to pay attention. By the mid-1970s, 2.5 million Americans were being diagnosed with a heart-related illness each year; 800,000 of those illnesses proved fatal. Heart disease accounted for about half of all deaths in the U.S. Speaking before the committee in 1976, Senator McGovern stated confidently, "Six of the ten leading causes of death in the United States have been connected to diet." Expert testimony led the committee to an inescapable conclusion: a diet high in saturated fats—such as those contained in animal products—was associated with increased levels of LDL, which leads to arteriosclerosis and heart attacks, as well as to obesity, diabetes, and other illnesses.

Witness after witness came before the panel to stress the links between a high-fat diet, high cholesterol, and coronary heart disease. "Diets low in cholesterol and high in unsaturated fats enhance the removal" of LDL, Dr. Robert Levy, director of the National Heart, Lung, and Blood

Institute, told the panel in 1977. Dr. Levy then proceeded to show the senators a series of diagrams illustrating the constriction of blood vessels by cholesterol-heavy plaques. Many of the witnesses at the hearings also named sugar as a dietary culprit. Dr. Beverly Winikoff, assistant director for health sciences at the Rockefeller Foundation, testified that obesity, and the resulting epidemic in diabetes and coronary disease, could be linked to increased consumption of both animal fats and sugar. Several other witnesses highlighted the sugar in breakfast cereals as a prime culprit.

The experts were agreeing with a consensus that had been building for some time in the American medical community and the public at large. When President Dwight Eisenhower was struck with a heart attack during his first term in office in 1955, the nation was riveted by the details of his recovery. Following his doctors' advice, the president not only quit smoking and lost weight, but also adopted a low-fat, low-cholesterol diet.

Eisenhower's doctors were influenced by the work of physiologist Ancel Keys, whose research comparing diets in different countries demonstrated an association between saturated fat intake and coronary disease. Although the limitations of his work were criticized, Keys was featured on a 1961 cover of *Time* magazine under a vivid illustration of an overweight man on a scale, a diagram of a heart, and a banner that read "Diet & Health." The Tobacco Institute praised his efforts and even helped to fund his research. Though it may seem odd that an industry devoted to promoting cigarettes would allocate resources to issues of diet, a cynical explanation seems likely: encouraging this newfound national interest in the dangers of food could divert attention away from the dangers of cigarettes.

The American public was becoming increasingly concerned that what they were eating might be killing them. Senator McGovern cited the growing awareness of the ways in which diet influences health, along with the popularization of fad diets and dubious health regimens, as reasons for the federal government to take action.

What the advocates of dietary reform did not understand, and what the senators were not equipped to consider, were the consequences of drastically cutting saturated fat from the American diet. If consumers dutifully cut back on fat, they would have to replace at least some of the calories it contained with something else. Where would they turn?

Carbohydrates.

Chapter 8

Government guidelines led us to carbs

With the best of intentions, the McGovern Committee took an unprecedented action: it drew up a set of dietary goals to be followed by all Americans. For the first time, the U.S. government took a position on what its citizens should and shouldn't eat.

Dr. Mark Hegsted, a researcher at Harvard University, had a significant hand in drafting the committee's nutritional recommendations, *Dietary Goals for the United States*. He then went on to draft guidelines issued by the Department of Agriculture in 1980. In his testimony, Hegsted encouraged Americans to embrace the dietary principles that are still familiar today: "We should eat less meat. We should eat less fat, particularly saturated fat. We should eat less cholesterol. We should eat less sugar. We should eat more unsaturated fat, more fruits, vegetables, and cereal products, particularly those made with whole grain cereals."

Other experts, including Dr. Robert Levy, expressed doubt about redirecting the eating habits of the entire nation based on circumstantial evidence. But Hegsted was undeterred. He confidently pushed for decisive recommendations, stating that there were "no identifiable nutritional risks associated with shifting our diet in the direction that I have indicated."

While Hegsted and others talked about eating less sugar and more whole grains, what they actually proposed in the guidelines was altogether different. The new recommendations were in fact the beginning of a slow-moving disaster. Here are the goals, first issued by the McGovern Committee on January 14, 1977:

GOAL 1: Increase carbohydrate consumption to account for approximately 55 to 60 percent of the energy (caloric) intake.

GOAL 2: Reduce overall fat consumption from approximately 40 to 30 percent of energy intake.

GOAL 3: Reduce saturated fat consumption to account for about 10 percent of total energy intake; and balance that with polyunsaturated and monounsaturated fats.

GOAL 4: Reduce cholesterol consumption to about 300 mg a day.

GOAL 5: Reduce sugar consumption by about 40 percent to account for about 15 percent of total energy intake.

GOAL 6: Reduce salt consumption by about 50 to 85 percent to about three grams per day.

Read Goal 1 again: increase carbs to between 55 and 60 percent of caloric intake.

This was not a misprint. It accurately reflected the views of many health experts at the time. Mark Hegsted and committee staff wrote the following in the report to the American public:

"Bread is of intermediate caloric density, and a relatively good protein source. . . . Contrary to what most people think, bread in large amounts is an ideal food in a weight-reducing regimen. . . . There have been no studies that have found whole wheat flour to be superior nutritionally to white flour when consumed in a normal diet."

Dr. Hegsted, like several other witnesses, seemed to believe that the main disadvantage of white flour was the loss of vitamins when the bran and germ of the wheat were removed. If white flour was "enriched" with those vitamins and minerals after processing, he believed it to be nutritionally indistinguishable from whole wheat.

Notably, the committee did not emphasize vegetables or legumes in its recommendations. Grains were to be the source of the recommended increase of dietary carbohydrates. The government guidelines were effective: they changed what and how Americans ate.

As advised, we began eating more starch. A lot more.

Chapter 9

———

"Complex carbohydrates" is a misleading term that fails to distinguish rapidly absorbable carbs from those we absorb slowly

What neither our public servants nor the scientific experts who were guiding them took into account when formulating national nutrition guidelines were the crucial differences in the way our bodies respond to different types of carbohydrates. They definitely did not understand the nature of the new fast carbs that were being introduced into the food system. Even now, government guidelines continue to lump together almost all carbohydrates, except sugar, with some distinction for "whole grains." To get back on track, we need to understand what carbohydrates are and how they are used by the body.

Long-chain carbohydrates are chains made of glucose molecules, which are essential for life. Glucose fuels essential metabolic functions that produce energy and power our brains. The vast majority of carbohydrates in our diet come from plants and can be categorized into three classes: starches, sugar, and dietary fiber. Virtually all starches and sugar are easily converted to glucose, while dietary fiber is not, because human bodies don't make the enzymes to break the unique bonds that hold together the glucose molecules contained in fiber.

Plants store energy as starch. In their natural state, the starch molecules in grains are extremely long. Before processing, a single starch molecule might consist of over *one hundred thousand* glucose molecules, bound together chemically in a twisted chain. Our bodies have evolved to digest these chains and use the energy inside. First, we grind the starch with our teeth; then the enzymes in our gut break down the chemical bonds of the starch, reducing them to simple glucose molecules that can be absorbed in our intestines.

Unprocessed fiber is made by plants to give their cells rigid structures that can bear weight. It consists of very long chains of glucose, but our enzymes cannot break the bonds that hold the fiber molecules together, so they are absorbed much more slowly. Fiber can only be digested when it reaches our large intestine, where it is fermented by bacteria, producing short-chain fatty acids that can be absorbed.

Sugars are a much simpler form of carbohydrate. Table sugar (sucrose) contains equal parts of two simple sugar molecules, glucose and fructose. They are quickly broken down in the mouth and absorbed as soon as they enter the small intestine—they never reach the large intestine.

As the distinctions among starch, fiber, and sugar demonstrate, the length of a carbohydrate chain and the type of chemical bonds that hold it together make a crucial difference in how quickly these carbs are absorbed by our bodies. When we talk about the absorbability of starch, we are talking about the pace and degree to which it can be digested, and where in the body that digestion takes place. Absorbability is a crucial consideration when we classify carbohydrates.

Until the nineteenth century, sugar was expensive and rare in our diet, but today, this rapidly absorbable carb is available everywhere. Many people who try to lose weight already know to avoid sugar, but they may not realize that rapidly digestible starches, including bread, other baked goods, cereals, and many of our favorite snack foods have the same effect.

The Dietary Goals issued by the government in the 1970s did not reflect any of this information. Instead, all carbs except sugar were grouped together under the misleading heading of "complex carbohydrates." This is a term that should be retired, because it fails to distinguish between carbs that are rapidly absorbed and those that are not. That ambiguity has long hidden the true nature of carbohydrates.

Chapter 10

—

Today's ultraprocessed foods allow us to absorb more calories

On average, we avail ourselves of about 500 calories more daily than we did in 1970. This is largely attributable to the fact that processed foods make up as much as 70 percent of the average American diet. While they sport countless flavors, shapes, and sizes and are sold under various brand names, their essential feature is the same: energy-rich carbs that have been dramatically altered from their natural state. Their molecular structure has been destroyed, essentially making them streams of glucose. In most processed products, a predigested starch is combined with some highly palatable additive—generally sugar, fat, or salt, and often a combination of all three—which makes them irresistible to many people.

A food designer who has worked in the industry for nearly fifty years described this change to me as "a kind of metamorphosis over the decades—we have made food itself nothing but easy calories." He said that the food industry had removed anything that could stand in the way of rapid caloric absorption. "Mill the bran off the white rice, refine the flour, so it's very light and doesn't obstruct you in any way. Light, easy to chew, easy to swallow. Make it more compelling by adding fat and sugar and salt: the perfect caloric torpedo."

The contrast with the food processing techniques used over the millennia could not be starker. Professor Rachel Carmody, a human evolutionary biologist, has written that early humans may have met their energy needs by cooking, since our relatively small jaws make it inefficient to rely on chewing alone to break down food. By reducing the structural integrity of foods, cooking made their calories and nutrients easier to digest and absorb.

Traditional societies also had tools for grinding and pounding grains, which gave us flour, one of our first processed ingredients. But simple stone-ground flour bears little resemblance to the starches we encounter on today's supermarket shelves. If cooking and milling were early forms of processing, today's food manufacturing strategies are more aptly called ultraprocessing.

And that points to another limitation of the current food label. While it reveals how many calories are in a serving size of packaged food, it does not fully reveal how many calories you will *absorb*. The key information about the speed at which calories move through your system, and where along your digestive tract they are absorbed, is missing.

"How many calories you actually get out of your food

depends on how highly processed it is," writes Professor Carmody along with her colleague Professor Richard Wrangham. "Food labels ignore the costs of the digestive process—losses to bacteria and energy spent digesting." We absorb more calories, per ounce of food, from the processed grains in chips or puffed cereal than we do from the fiber in intact whole grains. Processing makes more calories available to our bodies, and that's what matters to weight gain.

"If you eat a starchy food raw, up to half the starch grains pass through the small intestine entirely undigested," the authors explain, discussing foods like potatoes. "Your body gets two-thirds or less of the total calories available. . . . The rest might be used by bacteria in your colon, or might even be passed out whole." This is the danger posed by processed foods: by destroying the natural structure of food, they short-circuit our digestive systems.

Chapter 11

———

The food industry claims there are no negative effects to processing

Of course, the food industry defends its processing techniques aggressively. I witnessed this firsthand in the auditorium at the Institute of Food Technologists' annual meeting. The organization is dedicated to, in its own words, "a world where science and innovation are universally accepted as essential to a safe, nutritious, and sustainable food supply for everyone."

The institute was giving a short course on food science, billed as a boot camp for people who want to learn about the food manufacturing industry. The narrative of trying to achieve a safe and nutritious food supply was certainly on display. Dr. Roger Clemens, past president of the institute, was speaking to several hundred people, and the subject of the talk was the role of processed foods in delivering nutrition. Dr. Clemens asked the audience if anybody liked Italian food. He warned that we would be better off opening a can of sauce, rather than simmering tomatoes in a cast-iron skillet, which, he said, leaches iron alluvia into the food. Clemens's suggestion that store-bought marinara sauce was safer than what we might cook at home was part of his larger argument about the benefits of food technology.

It was also a way to mock how any food can be made to sound frightening. Dr. Clemens argued that if he showed you all the toxicants in food that occur naturally, you wouldn't eat. In his view, any concern about food processing and food contamination was overwrought and misplaced.

Dr. Clemens grouped all forms of processing together, defining them in a slide as "deliberate practices used to change raw plant and animal products into food products we can eat." Under that definition, he could argue that what manufacturers do to food is essentially no different from what we do at home by washing, chopping, heating, blanching, mixing, or freezing food, except that manufacturers do it in larger volumes.

He asked the audience what the difference was between preparing and processing. His answer: scale.

Food industry experts like to present their trade as a force for nutritional good. After all, food technology has given us gluten-free crackers, lactose-free milk, spreads with plant sterols that promote heart health, and flash-frozen string beans. Not surprisingly, what the industry deems as healthy always seems to be the more processed product. In its view, fresh is not always best. According to the International Nut and Dried Fruit Council, for example, the antioxidant content of dried fruit is much higher than fresh fruit because "the antioxidants are concentrated in a smaller volume during dehydration."

Seeds, another form of fresh food widely prized by nutritionists, also earned Dr. Clemens's ridicule: he asked if we were birds. He asserted that we don't have the machinery to break down the seed shell, which is mostly cellulose, and thus the seed passes right through our bodies, resulting in no nutritional value. The advantage of processing, Clemens claimed, is that it does the chewing for you. People like processing, he said, for without it there is less variety and food would spoil.

He pointed to bread as another example of technology's value. When chemicals like BHA, BHT, and TBHQ were used to keep bread soft, people were able to store the loaf in a breadbox, he said. Then what he called scare tactics about the use of preservatives came along and these chemicals began to be used less often. That meant that bread had to be stored in the refrigerator or freezer to prevent it from becoming moldy. Dr. Clemens implied that this was outrageous.

Increased food availability, choice, affordability, and convenience were all benefits of a modern food system. He pointed to other advantages that might be even greater. Technology, according to Dr. Clemens, allows us to reduce the risk of certain types of health conditions and improve overall health, not the other way around.

He went on to decry the food classification system used by the United Nations, called NOVA, which aims to identify ultraprocessed foods and drinks. Scientists have singled out such products as threats to public health worldwide. "These are not modified foods," as researchers at the University of São Paulo have written, "but formulations mostly of cheap industrial sources of dietary energy and nutrients plus additives. . . . Ultraprocessed products are made to be hyper-palatable and attractive, with long shelf-life. . . . Their formulation, presentation, and marketing often promote overconsumption."

Dr. Clemens apparently recognized a significant threat to the food industry in a system that wants to classify food based on processing. He expressed concern that there is a movement under way in certain countries—a freight train, as he called it—to so classify food. Dr. Clemens made it very clear that he did not want to do anything to compromise the food supply but clearly thought that this classification effort needed to be derailed.

After listening to some of his other talks, I know that he believes that both fresh and processed foods are important in everyone's healthful diet. Yet the industry spends billions of dollars designing and marketing processed foods.

A food industry playbook lays out other messaging strategies. The industry understands and manipulates the public's skepticism and confusion about nutrition and confronts it by, in its own words, trying to "reset" and "reframe" the conversation.

For example, marketing experts know that consumers are trying to limit their intake of sugars. These marketers also recognize that urging us to be "moderate" in our food choices only "reinforces the sense of harm" associated with some of those foods. They instead try to convince us that healthy living is about "balance" and getting all the nutrients we need from a variety of food groups.

On the surface, the industry's focus on balance has appeal. If calories from sugars and starches affected our bodies in the same way as calories from spinach and broccoli, the industry's argument would have merit. But as we have come to understand, not all calories are created equal.

Chapter 12

From whole grain to the cereal box:
What are we really eating?

Walk with me down a field of wheat and look closely at those stalks, the amber waves of grain so central to the American story. Now, zero in on a single stalk and travel up the stem to the head of the plant. Observe the spike that tops the plant, with the cluster of spikelets attached to it. Each spikelet holds a kernel of wheat, also known as the wheat berry or caryopsis. This single-seeded kernel provides the source material for breads, cereal, and a vast array of other products in the modern food supply.

The outer, protective layer is the bran, where most of the insoluble dietary fiber is found. At the bottom is the nutrient-rich germ, the "embryo" of the seed, comprising about 2.5 percent of the kernel by weight. It is, at least in relative terms, high in fat. In the middle of that kernel is the dense endosperm, the built-in food for the plant embryo. The endosperm is composed primarily of starch but also contains some protein and accounts for more than four-fifths of the kernel's volume. All three parts of the kernel contain trace minerals and some vitamins. This structure is not unique to wheat: rice, oats, barley, corn, and many other grains have starch-storing kernels with similar characteristics.

We would break our teeth if we tried to bite into the hard wheat kernel. Instead, we have developed milling processes that allow us to break it open, giving us access to the starch it contains in a more digestible form. White flour is made from grinding and sieving the grain to separate the bran and germ from the endosperm. Most whole wheat or "whole grain" products sold today use this same basic process and then add back the bran, giving the product its appealing coloration, and perhaps some greater degree of firmness, and changing the flavor and texture. A true whole grain, however, is one in which the endosperm, bran, and germ are never separated out. This preserves what scientists call the food matrix, or the original molecular structure of a food.

Inside the natural matrix of the starch granule are glucose molecules packed tightly together in a semicrystalline state. Under certain types of microscopes, the crystalline chains resemble a cross. These areas are difficult for water and enzymes to penetrate, which helps make the starch difficult to digest and slow to absorb. Even when parts of the kernel are ground up during milling, the structure of the starch remains intact. The granules do disperse in a process called gelatinization, becoming easier to digest when the bread is baked. But that's a far cry from what happens during food processing today.

Chapter 13

Food processing changes the chemical structure of starch

Grains are no longer ground by large stones powered by water wheels, as they were in the not-so-distant past, but instead are milled by high-speed steel rollers. Although this milling disrupts the tight, compact bonds of starch granules, it doesn't dramatically transform them. It is a second step, called *extrusion cooking*, that upends the granules, pulverizing the amylose and amylopectin chains that contain glucose molecules. These processes result in *dextrinization*, the fragmentation of the starch molecule into chains of shorter length, which enables faster absorption in the small intestine. (One of my scientific colleagues told me that some extruded starches can be absorbed even faster than that great American invention, Wonder Bread.) Glance at many food labels and somewhere you will see the word "dextrose." That's a short-chain fast carb created by processing.

Cooking extruders, which transform every part of the

molecular matrix of starch, are widely used by the food industry today. Most of the grains in breakfast cereals are processed in cooking extruders, as are corn chips and other snack foods. Even the rye in many whole grain flatbreads is pummeled in extruders. The label on the package may claim that the bread is made from 100 percent rye and salt, but it doesn't say anything about how much the rye has been transformed. Extrusion is also used to create some of the vegetable proteins found in the increasingly popular vegetarian products designed as meat substitutes.

The attraction of such aggressive processing to corporations is obvious. The ultraprocessed powder that results is easily mixed and combined to make thousands of products. It's a classic example of "value-added" manufacturing that allows food companies to charge more for the same raw ingredients. Moreover, it's a way to create an aerated structure that delivers a desirable mouthfeel, or "pleasurable masticatory sensations," as Dr. Martin Scanlon, professor of nutrition at the University of Manitoba, explained to me.

Developed in the 1940s, extrusion cooking uses both thermal and mechanical techniques to process ingredients for cereal and many other types of food. After the endosperm of the wheat kernel is milled into powder, the resulting flour is poured as a stream into a tube or barrel at the back of the extruder. A stream of water is added for hydration, and other ingredients are likely to be added for flavor. Rotating screws blend the ingredients, producing the shear force that twists bits of starch molecules in opposite directions to fragment them. Intense pressure, sometimes exceeding one hundred times atmospheric pressure, forces the resultant mix up and down the tube, where it is kneaded over and over again.

The initial mixing is done in a cold environment, but the pulp is soon pushed into the heating section, where temperatures can exceed 300°F. The heat and moisture, coupled with the shear force, lead to gelatinization—the destruction of the semicrystalline structure that characterizes unprocessed starch granules. The amylopectin component of the granule swells, its molecular chains break apart, and the amylose leaches out. Additional heating and shearing promote further swelling and leaching of the starch.

Now in paste form and still under extreme pressure, the mixture is moved toward the front of the machine, where it is extruded through a die. If an O-shaped breakfast cereal is being processed, for example, it passes through a circular die. Once the molten product is released from the tube, the pressure suddenly plummets and the liquid within vaporizes, causing a massive expansion of the surface area. It is now in a highly viscous, plastic-like state, and it quickly hardens into a solid that will eventually become your breakfast.

The effect of these processes on the food structure and our metabolism has never been adequately studied. According to the scientist with whom I spoke, when they entered the extruder, the amylose chains had a molecular weight between 10^5 and 10^6, while the amylopectin weighed approximately 10^8 to 10^9. The weight of starch molecules as they emerge from the extruder will vary, depending on the temperature and pressure within the machine. The higher the speed of the rotating screws and the greater the shear force, the more fully the starch granule will have been degraded. While the final molecular weight varies, it can drop between 10^3 and 10^5. From a practical standpoint, these processes increase how quickly we digest these foods.

Other food processing techniques likewise lead to starch degradation, albeit to different extents. For example, General Mills is proud of gun puffing, which it calls the "key invention" that made Cheerios possible. For decades, Cheerios were cooked under steam pressure and then gun-puffed in separate machines. The technique has been tweaked over time, but the fundamental principles remain unchanged. Air is applied with great force, dramatically altering the product's shape and texture. *Fortune* magazine described the invention in the 1940s: "Going into the forty guns which look like heavy steel barrels, the cereals are damp and soggy. The barrels are clamped shut and revolved as the heat and pressure in them slowly rise. When the pressure has reached about 100 pounds, a workman flips the gun over, aims it at a wire screen and pulls a trigger. The gun goes *boom!* and a shower of Kix or Cheerioats hits the screen like hail."

After extrusion and puffing, the mix is ready to be cut, dried, coated, packaged, and shipped off to stores. The physical properties of the original starch molecule are no longer the same. The granule structure has been destroyed, the glucose polymer chains have been reduced in size, and their surface area has expanded, which increases how fast we absorb these foods from our digestive tract into our bloodstream.

———

The altered structure of processed starch makes it a rapidly absorbable fast carb

The physical and chemical structure of a food determines how quickly it will be digested and absorbed by our bodies. Simply put: the more fully the food matrix is destroyed, the more rapidly starch becomes available to the body as glucose.

The food processing industry's techniques for breaking down starch granules, whether through extrusion cooking, gelatinization, dextrinization, or other methods, have a common result: they speed up digestion and absorption. The only difference is one of degree. Extrusion, for example, produces a starch so shorn of structure that it is essentially predigested. Other processing techniques may not be quite as dramatic, but they are still sufficiently powerful to produce fast carbs.

Dr. Bruce Hamaker is a professor of food science at

Purdue University who studies the effect of processing on carbohydrate absorption. Although he acknowledged that various processing techniques degrade starch to differing degrees, the end result is almost always faster hydrolysis— that is, a speedier breakdown of the starch granule. "We're interested in the digestion rate of starch and the factors that affect how fast starch is hydrolyzed and glucose is released and then absorbed into the body," Dr. Hamaker told me.

Our bodies evolved and adapted to extract glucose from intact food, he explained. That survival mechanism may help to explain the startling size of our intestines, which are typically some twenty-five feet in length. "Long enough to get most of the glucose out of the starch, even if it's in a matrix," Dr. Hamaker said.

Today's rapidly digestible processed foods are available to the body well before having traveled the full length of those intestines. At Lund University in Sweden, Professor Inger Björck agreed that while the degree of processing is a paramount influence on starch digestibility, the choice of processing techniques results only in shades of difference. "Many of the processing methods that we utilize render the starch easily available," she said. "We have such an overwhelming overcapacity to digest and absorb starch."

Professor Björck, too, emphasized that what really affects digestion and absorption is the structure of the intact food. "The type of available carbohydrates, the way you present them to your gut, and the type of dietary fiber is very important" for how the body responds, she explained.

Vegetables are a good example of a starch that is generally absorbed slowly. In vegetables like broccoli or spinach, the cell wall structure is robust, primarily composed of the dietary fiber cellulose. The polymer chains in cellulose are connected by beta 1,4 bonds, which humans do not have the enzymes to process. What that bit of chemistry means is this: we can't break down and absorb this type of fiber until it moves lower into the colon or large intestine, where bacteria do the work for us, breaking down the cellulose and making digestion possible.

Traditional dietary recommendations emphasize the nutrient content of vegetables as their most important benefit. And certainly, their rich package of vitamins and minerals is valuable. Yet what vegetables lack—namely, their relatively low levels of starch—may be equally important. Unlike grains, most vegetables consist primarily of water. Carrots contain only about 12 percent dry matter while broccoli is almost 11 percent dry matter. Endive, head lettuce, spinach, eggplant, squash, and bell peppers all contain less than 10 percent dry matter. There are, of course, some high-starch vegetables, notably root vegetables or tubers, such as yams and white potatoes, which are 22 to 31 percent dry matter, but those are the exceptions.

Most of the time, when we eat vegetables, the food structure remains relatively intact. Due to both the intact structure of vegetables and their fiber content, we don't absorb all the calories they contain. The energy of unprocessed foods remains within a tight structure that our enzymes can't break down, so our bodies digest the food but don't absorb the calories.

The more processed the starch, the faster the food

remnants are digested. This is the result of rapid hydro-lyzation caused by the degree of dextrinization the starch has undergone in processing. The more processed the food, the faster it will be digested.

While it's true that, as the food processing industry argues, humans have always processed food, traditional techniques did not alter the structure of the starch granule to the same degree. In cereals that have simply been ground through roller presses, for example, the starch is not completely broken down and so it is absorbed more slowly by the body. It is the contemporary industrial processing that produces rapidly absorbable fast carbs.

Chapter 15

———

Processed fast carbs serve as delivery vehicles for the pleasures of sugar, fat, and salt

In *The End of Overeating*, I examined in great detail what happens when the first bite of highly palatable food lands on your tongue, immediately activating the brain's reward center. Some of the brain's circuits have already responded before you taste the food, thanks to visual and olfactory cues that trigger memories of the last time you ate something so tasty.

Recent research on the causes of obesity returns again and again to the role of neurobiology. A wide body of evidence demonstrates that highly palatable foods disrupt our body's innate system of appetite regulation. Eating hamburgers, pizza, milkshakes, fries, and other fast foods triggers the release of brain chemicals like dopamine, which focuses our attention on the experience of eating. The food itself effectively sends a command to our brain that says,

This is important; pay attention! Brain opioid transmitters further increase the pleasure that certain foods afford, compelling you to eat more, even when you're not hungry.

Food companies are well aware of the seductive nature of their products, and spend millions of dollars to create foods that trigger this neurological response. They also design food to achieve the optimal "bliss" point, the point at which it will maximize your pleasure. The net effect—the food you are eating captures your full attention and makes you want more—involves many of the same neural pathways as drug addiction.

When I wrote *The End of Overeating* I focused on the role of ingredients like sugar, fat, and salt in this process. I investigated the ways in which they stimulate the brain's reward center, especially in people who tend toward over-consumption or experience a loss of control around food. When I began to look at highly processed fast carbs, however, I was perplexed because starch doesn't taste like much at all.

Although it is a key ingredient in many processed foods, starch by itself is no more appetizing than the school paste we once made from flour and water. The term "white bread" has even become synonymous with bland or boring. Flavorless starch is certainly not something we are likely to keep eating for no reason. That raises an obvious question: What is done to starch to boost its palatability?

Gail Civille knows a great deal about how food is designed. An expert in sensory evaluation, she taught me that food is often designed to achieve the optimal "melt" in your mouth—intense but fleeting. When I called to talk to her about starch, she was a bit perplexed by my new focus. Starch isn't particularly pleasurable, she insisted. It does release glucose in your mouth, she acknowledged, but she said it was not clear how much we can taste it.

What use, then, is starch—those wads in my mouth that form as I eat processed carbs?

"I don't think you need it," she responded, "except if you want to sustain something in your mouth for a little longer." But as we explored the topic, we both came to realize that a bland wad of carbohydrate plays an essential role in delivering other flavors. "It becomes a good carrier for other components that are attractive from a sensory perspective," Civille said. "Starch is the backbone."

Starch, in other words, is a delivery device. Highly processed fast carbs are used by food companies as a palette for the rainbow of flavors designed to be super palatable. Starch is the canvas on which manufacturers paint sugar, fat, and salt. That may seem innocuous, but it's crucial to the way in which these foods offer pleasure.

Civille explained that though starch may be bland, people like the feel of it in their mouths. People don't like high-grain cereals, she explains, because we don't want all of these little particles floating around, getting stuck in our gums. A soft wad of starch sticks together and is easily swallowed, leaving your mouth clean and empty—ready, that is, for the next bite.

That bland wad of carbs serves as a barrier to satiety, because it literally melts in your mouth before you begin to chew. Chewing food is an essential part of the body's response to hunger, slowing down your consumption and giving you time to feel full and satisfied. When you swallow your food without chewing it, your brain doesn't get the same signals as when you chew. As a result, you are likely to eat automatically and continually.

Sometimes, highly processed carbs are delivered in a puffed form, crunching pleasantly in your mouth before they melt into a soft bolus. That sensory feedback gives people a lot of pleasure, Civille explains. "It's why people sometimes eat with their mouths open. The feedback is even louder."

Subjecting cereals and snack products to the high temperatures and shear forces involved in extrusion cooking gives them more air and crunchiness, Civille told me. Moreover, this kind of processing creates a greater surface area, exposing the product to more saliva and digestive enzymes, which leads to faster absorption.

Flavor, pleasure, and palatability are the messages the food industry is sending to our brains—and fast, rapidly absorbable carbs are the messenger they use.

Chapter 16

Without processed starch, we would not have a vast array of processed foods

Today, approximately 60 to 70 percent of processed food contains starch as its main ingredient. Wheat, corn, tapioca, rice, potatoes, and other starches have given rise to hundreds of thousands of products that line supermarket shelves and fill our plates in restaurants.

This plethora of starch products is quintessentially American, reflecting both the vast quantities of staple starches that are grown in this country and their cheap cost. Starch is used to thicken sauces, replace fat, improve mouthfeel, create gels and glazes, increase yields, encapsulate flavors, and preserve a product's stability and shelf life. As a corporate project leader from one of the nation's largest starch companies said, "We use starches in almost everything."

Yet food designers recognized early on the limitations

of natural starch that was not chemically or structurally altered. It was runny, had little versatility as a thickener, did not hold up well during industrial processing, and had an undesirable texture and a short shelf life. So, beginning in the 1940s, the food industry began to change the quality of starch with processing techniques such as extrusion, converting intact granules to more functional molecules. Today, a food designer has hundreds of modified starches from various sources to choose from when creating a product.

Different modified starches provide an array of textures, giving food the exact crispness, crunchiness, or lightness consumers want to experience. It is hard to underestimate the importance of the textural experience that flours and starches contribute to food. When a bread basket is placed in front of me at a restaurant, for example, it is not just the visual cue of the bread that captures my attention, but rather the ability to conjure in my mind the feel of that bread, including the chewiness of the crust. As a sensory experience that compels us to eat, mouthfeel is as important and powerful as sweetness and saltiness.

But whether they are used for their textural effects or the myriad of other qualities they offer, the modified starches on the market today all share a single physiological effect: when digested, they break down into glucose in the body.

Part III

———

Weight

Chapter 17

Recommendation: reduce or eliminate fast carbs for good to achieve and maintain a healthy weight

Whether we call them rapidly digestible starches and sugars, refined grains, ultraprocessed foods, or "ding dongs and donuts," fast carbs have taken over our diet. As I've underscored, reducing or eliminating fast carbs from your diet is the one simple change that will allow you to achieve and maintain a healthy weight.

Let's take a moment to detail some of the distinctions between fast and slow carbs. Fast carbs are rapidly absorbable and easy to overeat because they don't trigger feelings of fullness, or satiety. They are a primary ingredient in commercially available breakfast cereals; most types of bread, rolls, and pizza crust; many gluten-free foods; anything made with processed flour; and puffed or processed snacks, including a variety of chips and crackers. Fast carbs also include all types of sugar. Obviously, cakes, candy, ice cream, puddings, and liquid carbs such as soda, fruit juice, and beer fit this description, but once you begin to look for fast carbs, you will find them in numerous other foods too, often where you don't expect them, including in salad dressings, processed egg and cheese products as a substitute for gluten, and even some chicken and meat products.

In addition, some *unprocessed* starchy whole foods are also rapidly absorbable. These foods include white potatoes and white rice, which qualify as fast carbs. Exactly how quickly you absorb the carbs in these foods depends on how they have been prepared and how you eat them. Dr. Louis Aronne, a weight-loss clinician affiliated with Weill Cornell Medical Center, has shown that eating fast carbs at the beginning of a meal amplifies appetite and leads to weight gain.

Slow carbs, by contrast, include legumes and nonstarchy vegetables, such as leafy greens, cruciferous vegetables like broccoli and cauliflower, asparagus, bell peppers, and tomatoes. These carbs are high in fiber and contain only small amounts of starch. Legumes like beans, lentils, and chickpeas contain naturally "resistant" starches, so-called because the fiber around the starch renders them more resistant to digestion. The high protein content of some foods that contain resistant carbs also helps slow down digestion and makes them highly satiating. It is hard to overeat lentil soup or chili.

Likewise, certain grains contain starch that is absorbed more slowly than the starch in fast carbs like wheat. These naturally slow carbs include oats, barley, rye, buckwheat, and quinoa (which is technically a seed, but consumed as a grain), which also offer the benefit of decreasing LDL and other blood lipids and thus lowering your risk of cardiovascular disease. Rye has among the slowest absorption rates of any grain used in bread (assuming it has not been pummeled in an extruder), and buckwheat also contains many resistant starches. Certain forms of processing and cooking are especially valuable for preserving the physical barrier to digestion. Steel-cut and rolled oats, for instance, are digested and absorbed more slowly than instant and ground oats.

Some types of pasta are also absorbed more slowly in the digestive tract. According to Purdue University's Dr. Bruce Hamaker, who is one of the leading experts on how food is digested, pasta cooked al dente has a microstructure that entraps the starch granules. But this appears to be the case only in dried pastas made from durum wheat that was dried in cool rather than warm temperatures. Those pastas are firmer and have a stronger physical structure that resists rapid absorption.

Though fruit contains sugar, mainly from fructose, fruit also contains the fiber and micronutrients that are associated with improved control of blood glucose, blood pressure, and blood lipids, which lower the risk of diabetes and cardiovascular disease. Fruit juice, on the other hand, contains no dietary fiber; it is basically just liquid sugar.

Slow carbs do *not* include most products labeled "whole wheat" or "whole grain." These terms are generally meaningless and are used for marketing purposes; most products with this designation have typically undergone substantial processing that renders the grains anything but "whole." Dr. Christopher Gardner, professor of medicine at Stanford University, described having an epiphany when he understood that most whole wheat bread has the same effect on blood glucose levels as white bread. "It's powder," he explained. "There's no digestion left to do." Adding bran and germ to that powder amounts to a gimmick, with whole wheat bread becoming a mere "glucose delivery system."

This information is not generally understood by consumers, who generally identify "whole wheat" or "whole grain" products as health foods. In a 2018 survey that polled consumers about their food choices and purchases, 89 percent of people identified the supposed health benefits of whole grains as a reason for choosing whole grain products, while 41 percent of those surveyed identified taste as a motivator. Both figures represent marked increases from 2006, when only 32 percent of consumers chose whole grains for their perceived nutritional value, while 13 percent chose them for taste. This shift is not coincidental. The food industry sees "a new norm" in the public's embrace of whole grains and is promoting their value in commercials and on packaging. The uptick in the appeal of such foods can be primarily attributed to a growing population of health-seeking consumers, though the increase in those selecting these products for their flavor may be attributed to the added sugars present in some whole grain foods.

One major manufacturer has taken grain processing a step further, patenting a technique to make ultrafine whole wheat flour. This process reduces endosperm, bran, and germ to fine particles. This so-called ultragrain is made by grinding the "whole wheat flour to the particle size of white flour," according to the company's brochure. The company also claims to have improved the flavor by working with farmers to grow exclusive varieties of wheat that are sweeter than the standard variety. These characteristics seem to be a textbook example of a fast carb.

A look at legumes affords another opportunity to contrast the degrees of processing that can produce either a slow or a fast carb. Just as the wheat kernel needs to be milled before we can gain access to the starch granules, so too does the hard outer covering of a bean need to degrade for the seed to become edible.

Generally, beans are softened by being soaked in water and then cooked to the point of tenderness. The bean swells and gelatinizes during hydrolysis, but its thick cell walls limit the extent of those processes. Because the outer walls remain stable, the starch granules stay tightly packed within the cell, even during cooking. As a result, the surface area of the enclosed starch is not accessible to digestive enzymes. That structural integrity is an important barrier to rapid digestion during the journey through the GI tract.

But food manufacturers have plenty of strategies for turning the mighty bean into a fast carb. Beans can be subject to extrusion or another high-pressure process technique that degrades it into a starch with minimal fiber, ready for a swift attack by digestive enzymes. Take a look at the label for Black Bean Crunchers, a Nature's Harvest snack that offers a scant two grams of fiber in every serving (its first ingredient is yellow corn masa, followed by soybean oil, black bean flakes, and black bean seasoning). Likewise, two tablespoons of Desert Pepper Pinto Bean Dip (first ingredient: pinto beans) offer a single gram of fiber. Contrast that with the eight grams of fiber in a half-cup serving of canned black beans, and the consequences of processing become apparent.

One of the tools sometimes used to distinguish various types of carbohydrates is the glycemic index. This ranking system, developed forty years ago, measures the effect of a given food on blood glucose levels. Carbohydrates with a high glycemic index are rapidly absorbed, while those with a low glycemic index move at a more leisurely pace through the digestive system. People with diabetes often find the index useful as a tool for planning meals, but it is imperfect, partly because it measures blood glucose only at specific points in time after eating. It also fails to factor in the beneficial effects of foods high in fiber and the influence of carbs on gut hormones, which can increase satiety. The calculation also omits milk sugars, which don't affect blood glucose levels, or the impact of combining fast carbs with fats, which gives rise to the anomalous result that a serving of ice cream has a lower glycemic index than a carrot. While high-glycemic foods are generally fast carbs, low-glycemic foods are not necessarily slow carbs, as the ice cream example shows.

Research shows that measuring insulin levels after eating fast carbs is a better gauge of the effect of our metabolism than blood glucose. For example, highly processed, fine flour and less processed, coarser flour have the same glycemic index. Yet more refined flour has a much greater effect on insulin than less refined flour. The food industry has its own motivations for challenging the validity of the glycemic index, claiming it is unreliable as a guide because we eat meals comprising many different ingredients (protein, carbs, fats) and not individual foods. That's not a particularly valid argument, however, as rapidly digestible starches have a detrimental effect even when consumed with foods that contain more fiber, fat, or protein. The rate of digestion is proportional to the amount of fast carbs in the meal.

While the glycemic index may not tell the whole story, beware of high-glycemic foods. They are fast carbs.

There are other types of measurements that do provide a more accurate assessment of fast carbs, including the starch digestibility method, used primarily by researchers, which simulates the breakdown of starch in the GI tract and then measures the amount of glucose released over time. We can also compare the rise in blood glucose caused by eating any type of food to the level that results from consuming an equivalent amount of pure sugar. One notable finding from that analysis is that a bagel from New York City Bagel & Coffee House can raise blood sugar to the same extent as twenty-three teaspoons of sugar.

As these tools become more widely available and perhaps easier to use, they can be helpful, but for most of us, they are impractical for daily use right now. If we instead simply learn to identify fast carbs on supermarket shelves and restaurant menus, we take the critical first step toward addressing the real problem driving our struggles with weight.

Chapter 18

———

Highly processed carbs
wreak havoc on our bodies

To fully understand the damage these highly processed foods do to our bodies, we need to review the basics of carbohydrate digestion. First, a disclaimer: our bodies' digestive and hormonal systems are incredibly complex and even now are not fully understood. What I describe here represents a simplified version of what happens when you eat and digest food. Some of the complexities of this process are the subject of intense debate among scientists, and much of it is the focus of ongoing research.

For example, there is a growing awareness that our microbiome—the tens of trillions of bacteria that live in our bodies and with which we have a symbiotic relationship— plays a much more important role in digestion, metabolism, and overall health than previously appreciated. The full impact of these microscopic tenants is only beginning to be understood, but we are learning more each day about how a healthy and diverse microbiome can aid in digestion, protect us from disease, and possibly help regulate our moods.

But generally speaking, here's what happens after we bite into a slice of bread or a hamburger roll, a donut or a slice of pizza, a cupcake or a cinnamon bun. Any of these foods will easily absorb your saliva, forming a nice, soft paste in your mouth. By itself, this bolus is not especially pleasurable, as Gail Civille pointed out. But as we've seen, that wad of carbohydrate plays an essential role in delivering the fat, sugar, and salt that have been designed to make us overeat.

From the mouth, the bolus travels down the digestive tract, through the esophagus, and into the stomach. Normally, the grinding motion of the stomach and its acidic environment break foods apart, facilitating subsequent digestion. The feeling of a full stomach is one of the vital cues that tells our brains we are satisfied and can stop eating.

But fast carbs arrive in the stomach as a soft, porous paste. The stomach doesn't have to do any work to ready them for absorption. Instead, the wad of predigested carbs is passed on quickly to the small intestine.

The small intestine has three sections: the duodenum, which receives partially digested food from the stomach; the jejunum, which absorbs most of the nutrients into the bloodstream; and the ileum, which absorbs any nutrients that were not taken up earlier. As nutrients are absorbed, the small intestine allows them to cross the intestinal lining and travel into the bloodstream.

In evolutionary terms, the job of the duodenum is to

continue breaking down food through the release of enzymes. But the processing that strips a carbohydrate away from its protective shell turns a very long-chain starch into a very short-chain molecule. There is no need for the food to travel through the whole digestive tract. Instead, the duodenum easily breaks down the short-chain molecules into monosaccharide glucose, which is absorbed through the walls of the small intestine and released directly into the bloodstream.

By doing so, highly processed carbs short-circuit our innate biology. The laborious series of steps we developed over millennia to digest whole fruits, grains, and vegetables through the entire length of the digestive system is undermined.

What happens next is that this large infusion of glucose in the blood quickly triggers the release of insulin. There's also an earlier place where taste or conditioning can trigger a "cephalic" phase of insulin production. Cells in the duodenum release a hormone called GIP, which increases insulin production. Insulin signals the cells in your muscles and liver either to use the glucose as energy or to store it as fat. Whether you've eaten a tablespoon of sugar or a slice of bread made with processed carbs, the effect is similar: your insulin levels spike. In fact, when scientists study the glycemic index, they use pure glucose or white bread interchangeably for testing purposes.

Fast carbs flood our system with spikes of glucose and insulin. And because we are eating fast carbs all day long, these spikes happen one after the other.

Chapter 19

Where we digest carbs determines how our hunger is satisfied

Our digestive process works very differently, and much more slowly, when the food we have eaten is not a fast carb, but a slow carb.

Let's take broccoli as an example. We have to chew it thoroughly, and then our stomachs grind it up and break it down. When it exits the stomach, the starch in the broccoli is still attached to cellulose (fiber) so that when it enters the duodenum, the amount of readily available glucose is relatively small. Consequently, little of the insulin-stimulating GIP hormone, one of two GI hormones called "incretins," is secreted in response.

The enzymes in the duodenum do their work so that some of the glucose can be absorbed when the vegetable matter reaches the jejunum. Here, in the lower parts of our gastrointestinal tracts, the arrival of glucose and other nutrients triggers the incretin hormone called GLP-1. By releasing hormones to tell our bodies that glucose is being absorbed, cells in the lower GI tract send a signal that helps extinguish feelings of hunger and produce a sense of satiety. Drugs that are nearly identical to GLP-1 are highly effective in treating diabetes and often result in significant weight loss for those taking them.

One hypothesis is that if a food never arrives in the jejunum (because it has already been absorbed in the upper parts of the GI tract), it cannot trigger the release of this other incretin hormone, GLP-1, and our hunger "switch" is never turned off. Dr. Fiona Gribble, a professor of endocrine physiology at the University of Cambridge, explained it to me this way: "Taking too much of your calorie intake as rapidly absorbable carbohydrate is not so important in terms of the physiological response it *does* trigger, but rather is unhealthy because of the physiology it *does not* trigger."

In another body of research, Drs. Andreas F. H. Pfeiffer of Germany and Farnaz Keyhani-Nejad of the United States investigated why different carbs had different glycemic index rankings. What they found was that *where* carbs are digested can be more important than *what* the carbs contain.

To conduct their experiments, they compared table sugar to a sugar that was harder to break down (isomaltulose). Because it took much longer for study subjects to extract glucose from the hard-to-break-down sugar, it was digested farther along the GI tract. In the jejunum, fewer cells produce the GIP hormone, but many more produce GLP-1, the hormone that triggers feelings of satiety. Thanks to its stronger chemical bonds, the more intact sugar helped to generate feelings of fullness, rather than triggering insulin spikes.

Let me emphasize this: eating fast carbs prevents us from achieving a sense of satiety because they fail to stimulate the signals that should tell us we are full. Even though our bodies have absorbed the calories, our hunger is not satisfied.

What's fascinating is that the two incretin hormones, GIP and GLP-1, seem to have very different effects. As Drs. Pfeiffer and Keyhani have suggested, "GIP has mostly unfavorable, while GLP-1 has beneficial metabolic and cardiovascular properties."

As researchers are only beginning to understand, the intestine is not a neutral processing machine; there are a number of different sensors that detect the arrival of glucose. It's as if you have a second set of taste buds in your intestines. Your duodenum "tastes" the glucose and triggers the reward circuitry in your brain. The same neural networks that are activated in response to the taste of pizza or a cupcake in your mouth light up once again. Indeed, some research indicates that the reward response in the gut may be even stronger than that in the brain. Exactly how these sensors interact with the incretin hormones is still a mystery, but no doubt there is a connection between the incretin molecules and the gut-brain reward response.

Dr. Anthony Sclafani, a researcher at the City University of New York, has studied this response. He says experiments with rats have shown that once the glucose "hits the gut, the intestines send a very rapid signal to the brain that stimulates the rodents' appetite for that sugar." This causes the animals to want more, whether they are being fed pure glucose or glucose-containing sugars or short-chain carbs (including food additives like sucrose, high-fructose corn syrup, and maltodextrin). They are driven to keep consuming, he says, "because they're getting this rapid post-oral response." In other words, their guts—and presumably ours—sense glucose and send a signal to the brain commanding them to eat more.

This finding has been borne out in other animal experiments. For example, according to Dr. Sclafani, there is a strain of laboratory mice that lack taste buds for sweetness. When these mice are initially fed a drink containing glucose, they have no reaction to it because they simply can't taste it. But if they are given the sugar for several days, they nonetheless learn to prefer it because the sugar is stimulating the gut-brain appetite pathway.

Another of Dr. Sclafani's findings is even more intriguing. He fed normal mice two different drinks: a sweet, noncaloric drink (sucralose) and a less sweet caloric drink (glucose). These mice had intact sweet taste buds and would be expected to prefer the sweeter drink. Initially, they did. But over a period of days, they changed their behaviors, opting instead for the less sweet glucose drink. The researchers inferred that the mice were sensing the glucose in their intestines. This delayed response was stronger than the initial pleasure they had derived from the sweeter drink in their mouths.

We shouldn't just focus on where and how rapidly fast

carbs are absorbed. We also need to consider the fiber content of our food. If we are eating relatively intact carbs, our digestive system still has work to do, past the early sections of the GI tract. All the cellulose fiber, which can be half of the dry matter in vegetables, remains undigested after it passes down the GI tract. This fiber, with some residual long-chain carbs attached, moves on to the large intestine, or colon. Fiber is an important part of your diet, not only because it provides the bulk or "roughage" that you need for bowel regularity, but also because it is essential food for the bacteria in your microbiome. These microorganisms aren't helping us for free; they rely on us to supply them with food. Over the past decade, scientists have invested considerable energy in studying this relationship. Surprisingly, as much as 50 percent of the calories we eat may be consumed by the bacteria in our gut.

"When you measure the caloric exchange in feces, half of the calories in a given food are absorbed by bacteria, not by the host," explained Dr. Dariush Mozaffarian, dean of the Friedman School of Nutrition at Tufts University. "If you eat food that's minimally processed, up to half of those calories may not be digested by you at all."

We've seen that the hormones and sensors in our GI tract signal our bodies about what we are eating. Some scientists also suspect communication between our gut microbiomes and brains. As Dr. Mozaffarian says, "The gut microbiome communicates to the host through an array of signaling molecules that enters the bloodstream, and these appear to have widespread effects on a range of tissues that may include, directly or indirectly, the brain."

While the mechanisms of this communication remain a mystery, we do know that rapidly absorbable carbohydrates never become food for our bacterial guests. Instead, they are processed without triggering the natural signals that generate feelings of satiety. Reducing the amount of fast carbs we eat and consuming more fiber-rich foods can help us regulate the complex systems that govern appetite. And that means regaining control of our eating—and our weight.

Chapter 20

Highly processed food
triggers speed eating

Wanting to understand the link ultraprocessed foods have with weight gain, researchers at the National Institutes of Health (NIH) led by Dr. Kevin Hall launched a study to investigate this connection further. They recruited twenty adults, ten women and ten men, to live at the NIH for twenty-eight days. Participants were in their early thirties and somewhat overweight, with body mass indices (BMIs) ranging from 25.5 to 28.5. (A BMI under 25 is healthy; 30 and above represents obesity.)

Ten of the subjects were assigned to eat only ultraprocessed foods, and ten to eat only unprocessed, whole foods. After two weeks, they switched regimens. Both groups were told to eat as much or as little as they wanted and could eat for as long as sixty minutes at a time. The investigators attempted to match the ultraprocessed and unprocessed meals for total calories, energy density, macronutrients (carbohydrates, protein, fat), sugar, sodium, and fiber.

Unprocessed or minimally processed foods included fresh, dried, or frozen vegetables, legumes, fruits, meats, fish, grains, eggs, and milk. The group eating unprocessed foods also had unlimited quantities of snacks: fresh oranges and apples, raisins, raw almonds, and chopped walnuts. Recognizing the extent to which wheat needs to be manipulated to turn it into flour, the unprocessed diet included few wheat-based foods, instead substituting potatoes, rice, bulgur, and oats.

Here is a sample day's menu for the group eating unprocessed foods:

Breakfast: Fresh scrambled egg. Hash-brown potatoes (potato, garlic, paprika, ground turmeric, cream, onions, salt, pepper).

Lunch: Entrée salad made with avocado, onions, tomatoes, carrots on green-leaf lettuce. Olive oil vinaigrette, grilled chicken breast, baked sweet potato, corn (from frozen), skim milk. Apple slices with fresh-squeezed lemon juice.

Dinner: Stir-fried beef tender roast (Tyson) with broccoli, onions, sweet peppers, ginger, garlic, and olive oil. Basmati rice. Salt and pepper. Orange slices and pecan halves.

The ultraprocessed group had access to fast food, sugary drinks, snacks, chips, cookies, sweetened milk products, sweetened cereals, and sauces. A sample day's menu:

Breakfast: Honey Nut Cheerios. Whole milk with NutriSource fiber (added to ensure that everyone in the study received the same quantity of fiber, but not the same quality). Blueberry muffin. Margarine.

Lunch: Beef ravioli (Chef Boyardee). Parmesan cheese. White bread. Margarine. Diet lemonade with NutriSource fiber. Oatmeal raisin cookies.

Dinner: Steak (Tyson). Gravy (McCormick). Mashed potatoes (Basic American Foods). Margarine. Corn (canned, Giant). Diet lemonade with NutriSource fiber. Low-fat chocolate milk (Nesquik) with NutriSource fiber.

Volunteers eating the ultraprocessed foods hardly had to chew. Most of their diet was soft, its color palette ranging from white to beige or pale yellow. Starch was the main ingredient in many of their foods: muffins, cookies, bread, flour tortillas, and bagels. Less obvious starches showed up as thickeners and stabilizers in products such as gravy and canned ravioli. Their daily snack choices were of the variety familiar to any airplane traveler: packages of baked potato chips, cheese-and-peanut-butter crackers, Goldfish crackers, and plastic containers of applesauce.

Perhaps not surprisingly, the ultraprocessed group ate more than the unprocessed group. Participants gained about two pounds on the ultraprocessed diet and lost about two pounds on the unprocessed diet. Fasting glucose blood measurements, which are drawn on an empty stomach, fell among the unprocessed group and stayed about the same for those on the ultraprocessed diet.

Most interesting, though, were changes on the hormonal level. Among those eating unprocessed food, levels of the appetite-suppressing hormone PYY increased, while the hunger-signaling hormone ghrelin decreased. The unprocessed diet also led to reductions in adiponectin, a protein hormone that regulates glucose levels and fat metabolism. A protein related to coronary artery disease, called high-sensitivity CRP, likewise decreased. Total cholesterol went down, as did fasting insulin levels that corresponded to the decreases in blood glucose.

Perhaps the most remarkable aspect of these findings is that these differences occurred in just two weeks.

In the controlled environment of the NIH clinical center, the average person on the processed diet ate about 250 more calories of rapidly absorbable carbohydrates and nearly 250 more calories of fat every day compared to those on the unprocessed diet. It may or may not be a coincidence that these numbers are virtually identical to the average increase in per capita food intake over the past fifty years.

What is it about ultraprocessed foods that results in the consumption of these extra calories?

The NIH study's lead researcher, Dr. Hall, pondered that question at Nutrition 2019, an international conference of clinicians, researchers, and nutritionists. The composition of the unprocessed and ultraprocessed meals was comparable on many parameters, and participants rated both diets equally palatable and familiar, so those factors didn't offer a clue.

What did matter was the speed of consumption. A dietitian documented the time in which subjects finished each meal and calculated how much they had eaten and at what rate. The conclusion: subjects ate the processed foods much faster than the unprocessed foods.

"The ultraprocessed foods are much softer and probably easier to chew and swallow, and that might translate into this increased eating rate," suggested Hall, noting that the diets were matched for their calories, macronutrients, sugar, sodium, and fiber, but not their oral-sensory properties.

Speed eating is no accident. The food industry designs food to go down in a whoosh. A patent application to produce corn chips that are as friction-free as potato chips makes this clear. The patent specifies the desired textural attributes: crispness, crunchiness, and lightness. The challenge in meeting those goals is that conventional corn chips and tortilla chips are "undesirably gritty." The thicker cell walls of corn make these snack foods slower to break down as we chew, and they do not melt in our mouths. Like the potato chips and Goldfish crackers that were included among the ultraprocessed snacks in the NIH study, the new corn chips would achieve a high degree of "mouthmelt." They would disappear into the gut much faster than fresh fruit, raisins, or nuts, all snacks that actually require us to chew.

Light in the hand, the "improved" corn chip is crisp without being hard in the mouth and crunchy but not gritty in the gut. Producing that structure begins with crushing the kernels into minute particles. In a separate step, starch is cooked in water and similarly pulverized, and the corn and starch are comingled and fed into extruders that break down the grain's structure into "a highly gelatinized plasticized mass." The resulting starch is a pale imitation of its molecular ancestor. Almost pre-chewed, it is quickly dissolved, swallowed, and absorbed in the upper GI tract, never reaching the colon. The gelatinous mass might have imparted "a distinct fresh roasted taste to corn chips and a toasted taste to wheat chips," as the industry boasts, but satiety never sets in no matter how many chips are consumed. Rather, we consume chip after chip after chip.

Chapter 21

────

Eliminating as many fast carbs as you can is essential to weight maintenance

I am the first to admit that abstaining from fast carbs is very challenging, and the reality is that none of us are going to achieve our goal of eliminating them altogether. For me, the closest I can come to cutting them out of my diet entirely, the better off I am, because that's what keeps my eating habits under control. Other people will do better by cutting back on their consumption. It's critical that you feel comfortable with your own choice and draw your own lines, so that you can stick with a better diet over the long haul. But it's equally important to recognize that our bodies just can't handle the harms that fast carbs are causing.

Let's look at three studies, conducted decades apart, that point to fast carbs not only as the culprit in weight gain, but also as a key reason why most of us eventually regain any weight that we manage to lose.

The first study was done by a pioneer in the field of

obesity, Dr. George Blackburn, at Harvard. In the 1970s, Dr. Blackburn and his colleague Dr. Bruce Bistrian studied the effectiveness of low-carbohydrate, high-protein diets. They prescribed a highly restrictive, near-starvation diet of no more than 800 calories of protein and fat a day to patients who were trying to lose weight. After following hundreds of people, they compiled results that were fairly conclusive: they found that following a low-carb diet was a safe and effective strategy for weight loss. In their study, nearly all of their participants lost twenty pounds, and about half lost forty pounds.

This protein-and-fat diet was a radical departure from what was then the standard weight-loss regimen, a somewhat less restrictive diet of about 1,200 calories a day that included fruits and vegetables. That diet worked, too: patients lost weight.

As these findings suggest, those who maintain a rigorous and disciplined approach to eating over a limited period of time will lose weight. The danger typically comes once we reach our goals: after achieving a healthy weight, we begin to loosen our approach. In trying to transition from weight loss to weight maintenance, we find ourselves struggling to maintain self-control, and the weight we worked so hard to lose reappears, almost as if it had a mind of its own. This profoundly frustrating sequence of events has long been painfully familiar to me.

Dr. Bistrian explained that when the weight-loss study ended, the researchers recommended that participants slowly add back to their diets some dietary carbohydrates, starting with vegetables, and then some fruit. But they found that this approach led participants to increase their intake of all carbohydrates and then gain back *all* or at least most of the lost weight.

A fair criticism of this study is that the investigators didn't know exactly what their subjects were eating after they liberalized their diets. That made it hard to know how much of their increased carb intake was made up of whole grains and vegetables and how much of it was made up of fast carbs. They couldn't know how many calories they were consuming. Without that information, it is hard to gauge the contribution that rapidly absorbable carbs made to the resurgent weight gain.

But a large-scale European study known as the Diet, Obesity and Genes study, or Diogenes, provides a more detailed look at the role of fast carbs in weight regain. The Diogenes study followed approximately eight hundred adults from eight European countries, all of whom were either overweight or obese, with BMIs between 27 and 45. They were put on a strict, low-calorie weight-loss program of protein shakes and some vegetables. After eight weeks, the vast majority had lost at least 8 percent of their body weight.

This is where the findings get interesting. For the weight maintenance phase, the participants were divided into groups, each representing one possible combination of protein and carbohydrates. That resulted in the following food plans: a high-protein, low-glycemic-index diet; a high-protein, high-glycemic-index diet; a low-protein, low-glycemic-index diet; and a low-protein, high-glycemic-index diet, or a "control" diet.

All of the diets included approximately 25 percent of their calories from fat. In some locations, participants went to centers where they could choose from a variety of foods. In others, they were given information about dietary choices and did their own food shopping and preparation. Although the individuals were not told to limit their calories, they were asked to try to continue losing weight or, at the very least, to maintain what they had lost.

Those on the high-protein, low-glycemic-index diet had the greatest success maintaining their weight loss and were most likely to lose additional weight, while the group on the low-protein, high-glycemic-index diet was most likely to regain the weight. Just as significantly, participants in the high-protein, low-glycemic-index group were most likely to complete the study, suggesting that they had the least trouble following their weight maintenance plans.

Another research project, called the Direct study, was made up of more or less captive subjects. The participants were obese workers at an Israeli nuclear power plant, and as is traditional in some parts of the Middle East, they ate their main meal at midday. Because of the difficulty of entering and exiting the plant, they ate that meal in the company cafeteria, which allowed researchers to control at least some of the food available to them.

The study enrolled about three hundred participants who were followed for two years. As in the Diogenes study, they were divided into groups, this time built around three dietary regimens. One group was fed a very-low-calorie, low-fat diet; the second, a low-calorie Mediterranean-style diet that included a modest amount of fat (primarily sea-food and lean meat, vegetables, whole grains, and olive oil); and the third, a low-carb diet with no calorie restrictions.

The conclusions closely track the results of the Diogenes study. The dieters who were restricted to low-calorie, low-fat foods lost the least weight. The low-carb dieters lost weight fastest, and were most successful at keeping it off, while the Mediterranean dieters took longer to lose weight, but eventually caught up with the low-carb group.

But then something intriguing happened. Having successfully lost weight, the low-carb dieters began gaining some of it back about six months into the maintenance phase, which was one reason the Mediterranean dieters could catch up with them. What went wrong?

Most likely, the weight regain can be explained not by the diet, but by the behavior of the dieters. Subjects in the low-carb group had no calorie restrictions, but were asked to keep their daily carb intake to no more than 4 to 6 percent of their total calories. When the researchers had them tally their daily intake after six months, they discovered that carbs actually represented a surprising 41 percent of what they consumed. Without being fully aware of it, the subjects had abandoned their low-carb diet and began gaining weight back as a result.

Even after being carefully educated by the researchers, participants drastically miscalculated their own intake.

Not having restrictions on their carb intake led them inexorably to excess consumption.

This certainly rings true from my experience. It's when we expand our carb intake that we start regaining the weight we lost. Whether the cause is the additional calories we are now taking in, their effect on fat accumulation, or how the carbs influence our appetite is an interesting academic question, but of little practical import. Adhering to a strategy that markedly reduces fast carbs—not just to lose weight but thereafter—is key to maintaining weight loss.

Chapter 22

Maintaining weight loss requires
us to eat less over the long term

I decided to take a comprehensive look at the clinical
studies comparing low-carbohydrate diets with various other dietary approaches, including traditional low-fat
regimens. I was specifically interested in ad libitum diets,
in which subjects are at liberty to choose their own foods
without having to meet a specified calorie goal. That, I
felt, was the best way to judge how these diets would fare
in the real world.

In one analysis of the published clinical studies, I found
seventy-four randomized controlled trials and asked a colleague to assess them for quality, using accepted scientific
standards. Only ten of them ultimately met the standards,
but that was enough to confirm my hypothesis. In the
majority of the studies, the low-carbohydrate group lost
more weight than the low-fat group, with the difference
reaching statistical significance. The low-fat group did not
outperform the low-carb group in any of the studies.

But the problem of weight regain invariably surfaced

with the low-carb dieters. Part of the reason for this can be attributed to the fact that we tend to liberalize our intake after successfully losing weight over six to nine months, even though we actually need fewer calories to maintain our new weight. There's one obvious but not so easy thing we have to do: we have to eat less. One advantage of cutting out fast carbs is that for many people it is easier to eat less when we are not consuming them.

Dr. Michael Rosenbaum, a pediatrician and professor at Columbia University, has made the issue of weight regain his life's work. I asked him why weight maintenance is such a struggle for so many people. As we lose weight, he told me, hormonal and metabolic changes make our bodies more efficient at regulating energy. It takes fewer calories, in other words, to meet our daily needs. "If you lose 10 percent of your weight, on average, the number of calories you require to maintain that reduced weight will fall by about 22 percent," Dr. Rosenbaum explains. This process is called adaptive thermogenesis.

To maintain a 10 percent weight loss, Dr. Rosenbaum has calculated that the average person needs to eat about 350 fewer calories a day. He has hypothesized that our muscles become more efficient after weight loss: we require fewer calories, for instance, to walk one mile. His recent research suggests that a reduction in certain thyroid hormones may contribute to this effect. This may not be true on a carb-restricted diet. Dr. David Ludwig of Harvard University has shown that people on a carb-restricted diet expend 300 kilocalories more than those on a fat-restricted diet. In any case, the drop in caloric needs almost certainly reflects interdependent changes across the endocrine and nervous systems. At the same time, our newfound energy efficiency (like having a smaller furnace) may also lead to increased appetite, which becomes a further challenge to sustaining weight loss. Whether our bodies sense they are in "starvation" mode or our brains' reward circuits are hyper-responding to food cues has not been sorted out.

The National Weight Control Registry research study tracks thousands of people who have managed to sustain significant weight loss over an extended period. The average individual on the registry has kept off about sixty-five pounds for six years. Dr. Rosenbaum looked closely at this group of successful dieters and confirmed his calculations: after factoring in caloric loss due to exercise, that group did indeed consume 350 fewer calories a day than a control group with the same weight.

Reducing caloric intake for the long term—eating less—is essential to maintaining weight loss. And while that seems like an obvious enough statement, it brings us right back to the imperative of eliminating as many processed starches as possible. We have already seen how eating fast carbs diminishes feelings of satiety, driving us to eat more. When we cut out carbs we also eliminate two major sources of extraneous calories—predigested carbs *and* all the sugar and fat that the food industry adds to that starch. If you avoid donuts to spare yourself from processed flour, then you also benefit by avoiding the fat and sugar they contain.

Chapter 23

Creating new habits can lessen
the appeal of fast carbs

There are times when all of us rely on food to change the way we feel, regardless of its nutritional value. We are using food as a drug when we binge, eat when stressed, or snack late into the night. The parallels between overeating and substance abuse are striking, undoubtedly because the neural circuits involved in our response to food and food cues overlap with those that are involved in drug addiction. As these mechanisms take hold, eating becomes fraught with regret and self-criticism for many of us.

Some experts believe that the circuitry governing appetite and satiety is even more complex than the reward pathways that lead to addiction. "The neurobiology of appetite continually takes us back to much more primal centers in the brain," observes Dr. Stephen O'Rahilly, a professor and researcher at the University of Cambridge, who hypothesizes that appetite is rooted in some of the oldest parts of the brain, in evolutionary terms. "The business end of eating is fundamentally very deep, and we share it with a salamander." Food, like sex, is one of the earliest drivers of reward, directing our attention and giving rise to feelings of desire in the face of cues.

One of the best ways to deal with the power that food has over us is to find ways to reduce the mental gymnastics required to maintain control over eating, especially when we are triggered by food cues.

I believe most of us understand what we should be eating, at least on an intellectual level. But understanding alone isn't enough. In order for change to be effective, we have to truly want to change—and that happens at an emotional level. Only when we can view fast carbs as not simply bad for us, but as something we don't actually want to put in our bodies, can we make new habits that are sustainable.

There are other ways to create better habits. Psychologists recommend the use of a heuristic, a process for problem solving in which you adopt and follow a rule that guides a quick and automatic response in the face of temptation. By reducing the number of possible responses, rules increase the chance of achieving the outcome you want.

Any rule that we can adopt to limit fast carbs, and in turn the number of calories we eat, is useful in weight loss. Over time, the goal is for that rule to become so ingrained in your decision-making that you don't have to think about it—"When I sit down at a restaurant, I will immediately tell the server not to bring me bread." Creating such reflexive rules prevents any ambiguity or stressful decision-making. By reducing the attention we give to distractions and temptations, we can, eventually, become oblivious to them. After a while, such rules simply become habitual. Free from anxiety, we can learn to sit down to a meal without being pulled by our neural circuitry to make impulsive decisions that are not aligned with our larger goals.

None of this is meant to suggest a joyless, draconian approach to eating. You don't always have to say no to the bread basket or avoid French fries every time. But the less often you eat them, the less you will find yourself craving them. In the meantime, you need a sensible set of rules and practices designed to reduce your exposure to as many fast carbs as possible, while allowing for the occasional and carefully controlled indulgence. In the end, there will still be temptation and emotional responses to food—I don't believe anyone who claims that they never experience a craving to eat fast carbs. But I know from personal experience that it is possible to set yourself up for long-term success.

Part IV

———

Metabolic Chaos

———

Chapter 24

Recommendation: to avoid metabolic harm, reduce or eliminate fast carbs for good

Now that we have a better understanding of the effects of fast carbs on weight, it's important to consider the long-term effects of fast carbs on metabolism.

While the breakdown of ultraprocessed carbs into absorbable glucose and other sugars has been well documented in the scientific literature, less fully understood is the impact of unrelenting glucose, over the long term, on our metabolism. What happens to the body when it is constantly flooded with glucose?

A few basics: as with fat and protein, both sugars and starches provide energy that fuels the workings of cells and organs. Beyond their caloric contribution, sugars and starches also set off a cascade of reactions in the body. As we've seen, when sugars and starches are broken down into glucose, insulin and other hormones are released in response. Insulin controls blood glucose levels in part by moving glucose into certain cells where it can be stored as fat. Insulin also affects how the body uses that fat and provides critical signals to the brain that affect both energy and appetite.

Insulin resistance occurs when insulin fails to produce appropriate cell responses. Initially, our body responds to glucose spikes by making more insulin, but in some people, the pancreas eventually wears out and stops producing insulin altogether. That is a key reason why the insulin response triggered by fast carbs is so important to understand.

The complex and powerful effects of excess glucose should not be surprising. Other than oxygen and water, no molecule is as important to all life-forms. Even the most primitive organisms have elaborate glucose-sensing functions. Recent evidence now suggests that increased insulin levels affect dopamine activity in the brain, which acts on the reward pathways to influence our behavior around food. In effect, insulin resistance leads to a dysfunction in how the gut and brain regulate the appetite.

According to Dr. David Ludwig, fast carbs produce more insulin than any other food we eat, calorie for calorie, gram for gram. "We know that processed starchy foods—white bread, white rice, prepared breakfast cereals, cookies, crackers, chips, sugary beverages; the starchy foods and also added sugars—tend to produce very rapid elevations in blood sugar and in insulin." He added, "Whereas unprocessed grains, grains the way our great-grandparents used to eat them—steel-cut oats rather than instant oats, quinoa, some of these ancestral grains—produce a lower impact on blood sugar. And even lower than that are most fruits, nonstarchy vegetables, and beans."

Dr. Ludwig emphasized that the large influx of glucose that results from eating processed carbs can be very damaging to metabolic health. "Rather than a gentle tide, you have this tsunami rushing in and out," he remarked. "That takes a toll on the body—meal after meal, day after day. . . . Fat cells are flooded with insulin. It's a recipe for type 2 diabetes, cardiovascular disease, cancer, and neuro-degenerative disease."

Several studies link diet to metabolic challenges. In one, conducted by researchers Drs. Mary C. Gannon and Frank Q. Nuttall, who have done seminal work at the University of Minnesota, subjects with mild but untreated type 2 diabetes were placed either on a high-protein, low-carbohydrate diet or a control diet high in carbohydrates. The ratios of macronutrients in the two studies were almost mirror images of each other: the high-protein diet was 20 percent carbs, 30 percent protein, and 50 percent fat, while the control diet was 55 percent carbs, 15 percent protein, and 30 percent fat.

Neither diet was designed to help the subjects lose weight, although those on the low-carb diet did lose a couple of pounds, on average. Instead, the researchers were interested in the effects of the two different meal plans on blood glucose levels. Distinct results were evident: participants on the high-protein, low-carb diet saw their glucose levels drop significantly, while those on the control diet saw no change. In addition, on the low-carb diet, people did not experience large spikes in glucose throughout the day.

Below you will see two sets of graphs from that study. Both track the blood glucose levels for participants over twenty-four hours. Graph A reflects the data from participants on the control high-carb diet, and Graph B illustrates those on the low-carb diet. In both graphs, the dotted lines indicate the levels at the start of the study, and the solid lines show the levels after five weeks.

In the control group, there is essentially no significant change to the participants' blood glucose levels over the duration of the study—but their blood glucose does spike three times during the day, presumably after meals. In the low-carb group we see a dramatic difference in glucose levels before and after initiating the low-carb diet. The "before" data show the same spikes as in the control group. But after five weeks, the average participant's glucose level is lower throughout the day, with only slight increases occurring episodically.

The next two graphs measure the levels of insulin in the participants' blood. Once again, the subjects on the control diet show no difference before and after five weeks, as Graph A illustrates. But in Graph B, we clearly see that after five weeks on a low-carb diet, the subjects' insulin levels do not reach the same peaks as they did previously. On average, their insulin production fell by 25 percent.

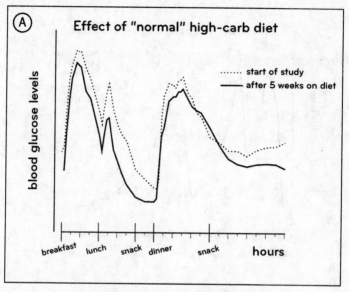

(A) **Effect of "normal" high-carb diet**

.... start of study
——— after 5 weeks on diet

blood glucose levels

breakfast   lunch   snack   dinner   snack   **hours**

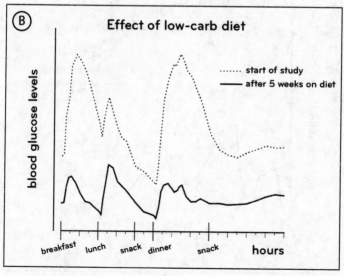

(B) **Effect of low-carb diet**

.... start of study
——— after 5 weeks on diet

blood glucose levels

breakfast   lunch   snack   dinner   snack   **hours**

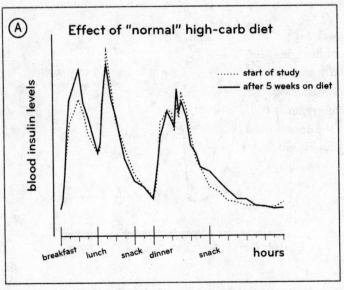

A

Effect of "normal" high-carb diet

blood insulin levels

.... start of study
————— after 5 weeks on diet

breakfast · lunch · snack · dinner · snack · · · hours

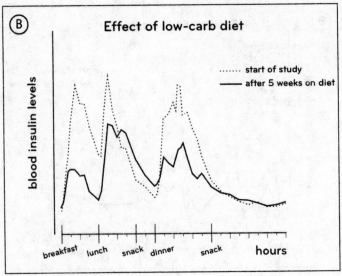

B

Effect of low-carb diet

blood insulin levels

.... start of study
————— after 5 weeks on diet

breakfast · lunch · snack · dinner · snack · · · hours

These graphs offer unambiguous evidence that reducing carbohydrate intake can decrease both blood glucose and insulin levels. According to Dr. Gannon, the evidence suggests that it is possible to reset the body's metabolic machinery in a short period of time with diets that contain what Drs. Gannon and Nuttall refer to as LoBAG (low-biologically-available glucose). Dr. Gannon recognized that their results were important not only for people with type 2 diabetes. "As we age, metabolism changes," Dr. Gannon said. "In order to live our healthiest lives, we have to try to adjust some of our lifestyle patterns. One of the easiest things to do to control blood glucose is to decrease the ingestion of starches and sugars."

While it's clear that lowering carbohydrates helps to even out glucose and insulin spikes, the quality of those carbohydrates—whether from whole food carbs or highly processed ones—also greatly impacts health outcomes, as indicated by several studies, as does cutting calories.

In the large-scale AlEssa study, researchers looked at the association between diet and type 2 diabetes in over 70,000 American women. Specifically, they wanted to examine the *quality* of the carbohydrates the women ate, rather than just the quantity. They assessed this by looking at the ratio of starch to fiber. A low starch-to-fiber ratio, such as that found in many vegetables, is generally a signal of higher-quality carbs (the slow-to-digest foods we call slow carbs).

The researchers in the AlEssa study relied on the well-known Nurses' Health Study, which surveys more than

120,000 female nurses from eleven states. The women have been tracked over the course of decades, beginning in 1976. Every four years, the participants have answered detailed questionnaires about their diet: what they ate, how often, how much, and so on. Examining this trove of nutritional data, the researchers asked whether the ratio of starches to fiber had any bearing on health outcomes.

The study considered a number of variables, including different types of fiber, but in the end, the findings were consistent. It wasn't total carbohydrate intake that was linked to diabetes, but rather a high ratio of rapidly absorbable carbohydrates to fiber. Women who ate a diet rich in highly refined and processed grains were significantly more likely to develop type 2 diabetes than those who did not.

Analyzed data from men came to similar conclusions. Research led by Shilpa N. Bhupathiraju at Harvard School of Public Health focused on the effect of foods with a high glycemic index, the measure of how quickly those carbs are broken down into glucose, and a high glycemic load, the indicator of the total quantity of carbohydrates in the food. Highly processed carbs have both a high glycemic index and a high glycemic load.

As in the AlEssa study, the Bhupathiraju group found that participants who ate diets rich in foods with a high glycemic index and a high glycemic load, and that were low in fiber, had an increased risk of developing type 2 diabetes. In some cases, that risk was as much as 50 percent more.

On the other side of the globe, findings from over 64,000 Chinese women showed a similar relationship between highly processed carbs and diabetes. Dr. Raquel Villegas of Vanderbilt University Medical Center led the research. As in the Nurses' Health Study, the Chinese women were followed over time and were asked questions about their health and dietary habits. Their diets were examined from different angles, including the carbs-to-protein-to-fat ratio, glycemic index, and glycemic load.

Once again, researchers found that the women who ate foods with a high glycemic index and a high glycemic load were significantly more likely to develop diabetes. Those who were obese faced an even greater risk. Someone who had both dietary and weight risk factors was at a 43 percent elevated risk of developing the disease.

Other studies have reached similar conclusions: the combination of obesity and highly processed carbs puts us on a path toward diabetes. A study of Japanese factory workers led by researcher Masaru Sakurai at Kanazawa Medical University in Japan found that when obese men ate a diet of more than 65 percent carbs, they greatly increased their chance of developing diabetes. Interestingly, in that study, eating a high-carb diet did not seem to lead to diabetes in men who weren't already obese. It's worth noting that these studies are observational in design and have limitations.

Nevertheless, these studies raise the question in my mind as to whether one segment of the population is particularly prone to obesity and diabetes. We may ultimately discover this to be so, and perhaps even learn what distinguishes the two groups. But on the basis of what we know now, the safest conclusion we can draw is that anyone who eats too many fast carbs is at an increased risk of developing significant metabolic disease.

Chapter 25

———

Consumption of fast carbs may lead to metabolic syndrome

Thirty years ago, American endocrinologist Dr. Gerald Reaven advanced the concept of "metabolic syndrome" to describe the host of symptoms that indicate the body's metabolism is malfunctioning. Metabolic syndrome can be a harbinger of type 2 diabetes, cardiovascular disease, and even cancer. As we age, our risk of metabolic syndrome increases.

Reaven hypothesized that insulin resistance was the underlying factor for metabolic syndrome. Associated with that insulin resistance is abdominal obesity, elevated blood glucose, elevated blood pressure, and increased triglycerides (a category of blood lipids). These unwelcome symptoms are associated with accumulation of fat around the liver.

Elevated insulin and blood glucose levels redirect excess energy by stimulating the production of liver fat. This lays the foundation for the development of fatty liver disease.

Two additional studies add support for the role of diet in developing metabolic syndrome. In one, scientists collected data from surveys of a Korean population that had been conducted annually from 2007 to 2014, and then analyzed findings from a group of over 38,000 adults. As in other studies, they had to control for many variables, including age, gender, and lifestyle factors such as exercise. The researchers concluded that women who consumed high-carbohydrate diets were at greater risk for developing metabolic syndrome than their peers who consumed lower-carbohydrate diets. Interestingly, increased fat intake was associated with a lower risk of metabolic syndrome.

In another study conducted in Chennai, India, scientists specifically looked at the effects of refined grains—in this case, processed or white rice. They, too, found that the incidence of metabolic syndrome tracked with the consumption of these processed carbs. Subjects who ate the highest percentage of refined rice were, on average, seven times more likely to develop metabolic syndrome.

There is additional very compelling evidence that starch is at the center of metabolic dysregulation. The evidence comes in the form of a drug called acarbose, which inhibits the breakdown and absorption of starch in the gastrointestinal tract. In a randomized controlled clinical trial, participants who took acarbose in combination with a traditional Western (non-low-carb) diet reduced their risk of diabetes by 25 percent, cardiovascular disease by 49 percent, and hypertension by 34 percent. A published analysis of all relevant clinical trials involving acarbose confirms these findings. While I believe this study offers very useful insight into the role of blocking starch absorption to prevent type 2 diabetes, I do not recommend taking a drug as a shortcut to eating a healthy diet. Acarbose should not be viewed as a safeguard or shortcut that allows you to continue to eat fast carbs.

Still more evidence about the effects of fast carbs comes to us from England, where two different diets were tested on a group of men: one was based on foods with a high glycemic index, the other on low glycemic index foods. The men ate one diet for a week and then, after a one-month pause, ate the alternative diet for another week. The researchers tested the participants for the effects on blood glucose and insulin levels, as well as for signs of fat around the liver. After just one week on the high glycemic index diet, measures of liver fat rose, while a single week on the low glycemic index diet caused these measures to drop.

As Professor Gerald Shulman, a world-class endocrinologist and my colleague from Yale, has shown, ingesting excess carbohydrates increases liver fat production by 40 percent and is accompanied by a doubling of new fat synthesis. That liver fat increases blood lipids and fatty acids, and thus the risk of heart disease. The spillover of fatty acids from the liver also results in increased fat storage in muscle and fat cells, which ultimately leads to fatty liver disease, weight gain, worsening insulin resistance, and diabetes. Here, the map of the causal relations becomes complicated, thick with arrows pointing in both directions. Fatty liver disease produces two types of lipid molecules in the bloodstream—triglycerides and LDL—both of which contribute to heart disease. Some have suggested that fatty liver disease precedes the development of both diabetes and metabolic syndrome.

Normal aging also contributes to this buildup of liver fat. The parts of our cells that are responsible for producing energy and burning fat are called mitochondria. As we age, our mitochondria slow down. When we reach our seventies, our muscle mitochondrial function is reduced by 35 percent from its peak in our twenties. This natural slowing of the mitochondria, according to Shulman, predisposes us to building up fat in our muscles, with concomitant increases in insulin resistance and diabetes.

The good news is that the gradual slowing of mitochondria can be countered by exercise. Indeed, this is why exercise is so important in preventing not only obesity but also metabolic disease. Professor Shulman has shown that even a single session of vigorous exercise can effect for the better the abnormal storage of carbohydrate as fat in patients with insulin resistance. Adequate exercise is critical to metabolic health. Indeed, research has shown that endurance athletes seem to be protected against insulin resistance because of their "high functioning" mitochondria. Exercise is a key tool to improve insulin sensitivity and keep us metabolically healthy.

Chapter 26

Fast carbs interfere
with fat metabolism

Processed carbohydrates become even more problematic when they are combined with fats. Ordinarily, eating fat turns on a master molecular switch (PCG-1 alpha) that increases your capacity to burn that fat. But eating glucose-rich foods suppresses that response, shutting off many oxidative pathways that convert these molecules into energy and restricting your fat-burning ability.

Dr. Brian DeBosch, who has studied these cellular mechanisms at Washington University at Saint Louis, can rattle off a litany of reasons why excess glucose interferes with weight loss. Chief among them is that it stimulates the protein switch that suppresses the pathways by which fat gets burned. The consistently high levels of insulin stimulated by that glucose also keep fat storage pathways active and interfere with our ability to feel satiated.

Dr. Elizabeth Parks, a professor at the University of Missouri who studies fat metabolism, put it more simply when I asked about the combination of fat and carbohydrates. "If you eat a pat of butter first thing in the morning, you will burn the fat. If you eat a pat of butter and a jellybean, which has sucrose and fructose in it, you will store the fat," she said. "Once the sugar has cleared and been made into fat, it broadcasts a message to the liver, 'Store any fat that comes to you. We're fed.'"

Along with that, she and I discussed how fat amplifies the rewarding effects of processed carbs.

While I will eat carbohydrates alone to excess, fat doesn't prompt the same overeating behavior. On its own, fat doesn't raise insulin, nor disrupt our system of appetite regulation. "Nobody binges on olive oil. Nobody binges on avocado. In fact, nobody binges on butter," said Dr. David Ludwig. But when fat is combined with carbs, excessive consumption becomes all too easy. Most of us aren't eating pats of butter off a fork, but use a knife to spread it on a piece of baguette, and before we know it, we've eaten half a loaf of bread and half a stick of butter.

There are varying points of view about the biological mechanisms that allow refined carbohydrates to contribute to metabolic disease and weight gain.

Dr. Ludwig believes that restricting carbohydrates results in an increase in energy expenditure—we burn more calories—and, by extension, experience greater weight loss. His studies have shown detailed evidence demonstrating that we burn more energy on low-carb diets.

By contrast, Dr. Kevin Hall, the National Institutes of Health researcher, believes that such carb-restricted diets may lead to less energy intake. Simply, we eat less by decreasing palatability, decreasing appetite, or increasing satiety. Dr. Hall disagrees with Dr. Ludwig as well about the measurement of energy burned. He points to studies that show there is very little difference in how much energy is burned. Some of the results from these same studies seem to favor lower-fat diets.

While the mechanism behind metabolic syndrome has not yet been identified, what Ludwig and Hall do agree on is significant: that restricted carbohydrate diets can reduce elevated levels of insulin in our blood known as hyperinsulinemia. Hall confirmed this in a conversation and added, "A whole host of things happen when you do this." He described an increase in the breakdown of fat (lipolysis) in the triglycerides stored in fatty tissue. Ketones, the molecule produced by the liver from burning fat stores in the body, also rise, although whether increased ketones themselves are beneficial is unknown. So, too, do glycerol and free fatty acids, which are components of fat molecules that either come from our diet or are produced in our bodies and then circulate in the blood. All of that means that more fat gets released from cells and burned as fuel.

Another researcher, Dr. Jeannie Tay, at the University of Alabama at Birmingham, has conducted several clinical trials that demonstrate the value of restricting carbohydrates and increasing intake of unsaturated fat. Her work shows that these steps can improve blood glucose control and markers of cardiovascular risk, even in the absence of weight loss.

Despite some differences of opinion among learned

experts, and important knowledge gaps that are yet to be filled, a body of pivotal studies is heading toward a similar conclusion: that highly processed food is problematic not because of some weakness in ourselves but because of the design and nature of the food itself.

Chapter 27

A vicious cycle connecting fast carbs, obesity, and diabetes traps many people who struggle with their weight

We now know even more about some of the roots of obesity and diabetes.

The hardest question that I've been asked is why certain people struggle to maintain a healthy weight and others do not. A possible answer came from Dr. Dana Dabelea, a professor of epidemiology and pediatrics, during a lecture at the International Diabetes Federation Congress in Busan, South Korea in late 2019. In her discussion on the prevention of type 2 diabetes, she presented data demonstrating that fetal exposure to diabetes was the strongest risk factor for developing type 2 diabetes in youth.

As a pediatrician, I was trained to think about the developmental origins of diseases, specifically how exposures to the fetus can lead to disease in later life. For several decades, epidemiologists have suggested that undernutrition during fetal life can lead to metabolic disease if the child is exposed after birth to an overabundance of food.

Dr. Dabelea's research looks instead to overnutrition and shows how fetal overnutrition increases the possibility of developing obesity and diabetes during life. The greater the mother's weight prior to pregnancy, and the greater the weight gain during pregnancy, the greater the weight later, in childhood.

Exposure to overnutrition is not only important during fetal development, but also during critical life periods such as puberty. Under these conditions, the body enters a period of insulin resistance. The logical but unfortunate consequence is that this can trigger its own vicious cycle of obesity and diabetes: maternal obesity and diabetes lead to fetal overnutrition, which results in adolescent obesity and early youth onset type 2 diabetes, begetting adult obesity, and, in women, maternal obesity and diabetes.

I asked Dr. Dabelea how overnutrition caused the later life consequences. "Overnutrition results from excess maternal fuels available to the fetus. The most important one, given our data, seems to be glucose," she said. "None of the other fuels, including fatty acids, which cross the placenta and contribute to overnutrition, seem to do the same thing."

If exposure to excess glucose during these sensitive periods sets up our biology for a lifetime struggle, we have a chance to protect the next generation. We need to be adamant that we question the quality of the food supply, not the mother. Women must have access to healthy whole foods both before and during pregnancy. Avoiding excessive fast carbs and processed food, providing good maternal care (not forgetting folic acid supplementation to prevent the risk of neural tube defects), and assuring interventions in childhood and adolescence may be the most promising strategies to prevent the intergenerational transfer of obesity and type 2 diabetes.

As we move further into the scientific frontier, the debate among experts becomes more intense. What exactly is the relationship between rapidly absorbable fast carbs and obesity and metabolic disorders, including diabetes? No responsible scientist doubts that these diseases cluster in the same individuals, but researchers still struggle to understand what is cause and what is effect. Like many questions in clinical medicine, the problem resembles a classic chicken-or-egg paradox. Does elevating blood glucose and insulin levels on a chronic basis cause disease? Or is it obesity itself that causes disease? The complexity of our metabolic pathways makes it difficult to arrive at an answer.

Typically, experts have assumed that diet drives obesity, which causes insulin resistance, which leads to hyperinsulinemia and damage to the beta cells of the pancreas, which is the key insult in type 2 diabetes. But Professor James Johnson of the University of British Columbia suggests that this is not the only possible model. He hypothesizes that diet might cause hyperinsulinemia, and hyperinsulinemia can then cause obesity, rather than the other way around. Indeed, he has shown that protecting against hyperinsulinemia can also protect against obesity.

The influence of diet may also depend on other physiological characteristics. "I don't believe that a high-carbohydrate diet causes diabetes in the absence of weight gain," says Dr. Ralph DeFronzo, a leading diabetologist. "But a high-carbohydrate diet is a *disaster* for glycemic control in a diabetic. These patients have a problem secreting enough insulin, including secreting it quickly enough. If you start feeding them a lot of carbohydrate, you're going to elevate the blood glucose levels and develop hyperglycemia."

On that point there is consensus. If an individual has diabetes, a high-carb diet is clearly damaging. But that doesn't tell us whether glucose can damage the metabolism of an otherwise healthy person, independent of weight. "The answer to that question is not known," Dr. DeFronzo admitted, but a body of accumulating science suggests that it may. DeFronzo described attempts to test the question by introducing large amounts of glucose directly into the bloodstream of study subjects. Researchers found that giving people intravenous glucose over seventy-two hours temporarily decreased insulin's effectiveness (insulin resistance) in their livers, and it seems reasonable to assume that, over time, eating foods high in glucose would produce similar results.

After three days of intravenous glucose, study participants did not show any sign of impaired beta cell function, the hallmark of later-stage type 2 diabetes. But Dr. DeFronzo believes it is only a matter of time until they do. If glucose levels are chronically elevated over an extended period—a week or two—he predicts that beta cell function will begin to degrade.

As I worked to understand just what we do know about the elusive mechanisms linking obesity, diabetes, and metabolic disorders, a letter in the *Indian Journal of Endocrinology and Metabolism* caught my attention. "Two models of obesity exist that describe its causation," the letter read. One model is driven by an excess of dietary fat, the other by highly processed carbs. The writer, Dr. Somi Sankaran Prakash of Christian Medical College, was captivated by the same question I was—is hyperinsulinemia or obesity the trigger for metabolic disease?

What especially drew me to his work was this sentence: "It should be borne in mind, however, that although the origin and causative factors may be different in various ethnic groups, once imbalance occurs, then a vicious cycle ensues in all these populations."

I called Dr. Prakash and asked him to explain more about this vicious cycle. Here is what he sent me following up on our call:

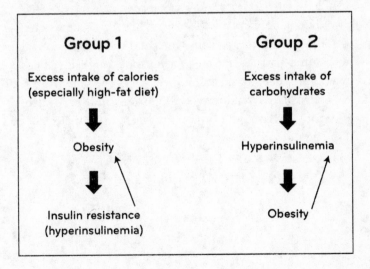

Food or Fiction?

For the vast majority of people, the sequence of the interactions isn't actually that significant. Whether excess glucose leads directly to insulin resistance, which then causes obesity, or excess glucose and fat causes obesity, which then results in insulin resistance, or if some other more complex set of interactions is involved, the solution is still to reduce fast carbs and the calories associated with them.

All this research is complex and rightfully generates fierce debate in the scientific community, which is reported in the press. I wonder whether that debate has wound up obscuring what is in plain sight: that fast carbs, obesity, and insulin resistance can easily entrap us and are linked to bad health outcomes.

Chapter 28

———

We have the ability to reverse metabolic disease

Not only can you stay metabolically healthy by eating fewer processed carbs, you may also be able to return to better health if you have already suffered the consequences of a high-carb diet. Hyperinsulinemia and insulin resistance are reversible, at least in some people. If you reduce the rapidly absorbable fast carbs in your diet, you can increase insulin sensitivity. This change appears to improve the brain's ability to detect satiety signals and ultimately affords more control over eating.

Dr. Ludwig has studied the clinical effects of lowering blood insulin levels by reducing intake of processed carbs and has found that reducing insulin levels is in itself metabolically beneficial. By contrast, he asserts, "When fat cells are forced to store too many calories, they outstrip their food and blood supply. They become necrotic and inflamed. Immune cells start to spew out all sorts of toxic interleukins [molecular signals], spreading chronic inflammation through the body." And inflammation affects a wide range of organs and tissues, including the heart and blood vessels.

According to Dr. Ludwig, when you lower insulin levels with a low-carbohydrate diet, fat cells can instead be prompted to disgorge some of their excess calories. That in itself reduces inflammation. As Dr. Ludwig explains, "Within three to five days, people with type 2 diabetes and long-standing high insulin requirements are showing remarkable remission."

"Five days!" exclaimed Ludwig. That's a truly dramatic pace at which to show such a powerful clinical benefit.

Here is what is happening: when we halt glucose intake, even temporarily, our entire metabolic landscape shifts. Reduce starches and sugars in your diet and free fatty acids become fuel for the body. Indeed, in a fasting state, these fatty acids are the body's major source of energy. "The glucose that comes from the liver is used almost exclusively by the brain," explains Dr. Ludwig. "A little bit by the kidneys, a little bit by red blood cells. Everything else is fueled by free fatty acids." These free fatty acids are not the source of problems—indeed, Ludwig calls them "our best friends."

Glucose, he explains, is "a messy fuel." Burning glucose is inefficient: it involves multiple biochemical steps and creates a lot of oxidative stress that results in more free radical molecules that can cause damage to our cells and tissues. Fat, on the other hand, is "a very effective fuel, just one step away from oxidative phosphorylation" and being turned into energy.

It is important not to think of hyperinsulinemia and excess glucose as issues only affecting those with type 2 diabetes. Tens of millions of people in the U.S. have prediabetes, or insulin resistance. For them, these biomarkers, such as their blood glucose level, may ultimately predict whether their conditions progress to full-blown diabetes. In addition, many people are living with the metabolic consequences of excess weight and accompanying hyperinsulinemia, even in the absence of prediabetes. About 70 percent of those with prediabetes develop diabetes.

Doctors who treat obesity and metabolic disorders are beginning to use these data in clinical practice. Dr. Jeffrey Sicat, an endocrinologist in Richmond, Virginia, described a shift in his own practice after he reviewed data from recent studies on diet and glucose control. This research showed improvement in blood glucose levels in just five weeks when patients switched from a low-fat diet to one that limited carbs to about 150 grams per day. (Note that this is nowhere near as low as the 30 to 50 grams recommended in ketogenic diets.) Many of his patients had been eating 600 to 700 grams of carbohydrates a day; reducing that number to 150 grams yielded dramatic reversals of diabetes risk. The takeaway is clear: cutting down your intake of processed carbohydrates even somewhat modestly can produce significant results.

Chapter 29

———

Improving metabolic health is important for preserving cognitive function, reducing the risk of certain cancers, and improving male libido

If the evidence I have shared thus far has not persuaded you to reduce or eliminate fast carbs from your diet, let me offer some final considerations. Because few bodily systems are spared from the metabolic consequences of excess fat—and fast carbs cause us to rapidly gain body fat—reducing fast-carb intake results in widespread health benefits. In particular, emerging science shows that improving metabolic health can lead to improved cognitive function, reduced risk of cancer, and increased libido in men.

Metabolic dysfunction increases our risk of Alzheimer's disease by 50 to 100 percent. The close association between type 2 diabetes and deteriorating brain health is well established, and when it is coupled with a family history of the disease that suggests genetic predisposition, the risk increases dramatically.

While the reasons for this association are still a mystery, some cutting-edge scientists probing the causes of dementia have identified numerous ways that metabolic disease may be implicated. The most likely link is the low-grade systemic inflammation associated with excess fat. Not long ago, the medical community viewed fat deposits in the body as relatively inert and assumed they did not generate much biological activity. But today, we know that "sick fat" produces damaging inflammation.

Some scientists have suggested that increases in inflammatory processes, as well as changes in blood flow, contribute to dementia. Others have suggested that the inflammatory effects in the gut microbiome may have an effect on the development of Alzheimer's by triggering the body's immune cells to cross the blood-brain barrier and generate inflammation in the brain. As we continue to explore this research frontier, here's what we do know: unhealthy waistlines and cellular aging combine to damage molecules and generate cellular debris and inflammation that can gum up our neural networks.

There is also a growing body of evidence that several cancers have metabolic roots. Elevated blood glucose and insulin levels increase the level of a key growth factor, IGF-1 (insulin growth factor), which is produced by the liver and facilitates the growth of tumor cells. That is one reason why obesity is considered a risk factor for postmenopausal breast, prostate, endometrial, and colorectal cancers.

Mutations in DNA cause the uncontrolled cell growth that characterizes cancer. That growth depends on cancer cells having the ability to continually divide, survive in the environment, and overcome any barriers that limit their growth. The insulin-signaling pathways that are triggered by "over-nutrition" support this process by activating genes that aid cell growth and proliferation. One example of the consequences is evident among women with early-stage breast cancer; regardless of their weight, this population faces a risk of recurrence and death that is doubled or tripled if they also have higher fasting insulin levels.

Male sexual function is also affected by metabolic dysregulation. In the early 2000s, several major pharmaceutical companies launched extensive promotional campaigns to market testosterone as a treatment for symptoms of fatigue and low libido in men in their forties and fifties. The companies tried to convince doctors and patients that the cause of their symptoms was a syndrome involving low testosterone blood levels, which they nicknamed "low T." Unfortunately, as use of testosterone replacement therapy rose, so did heart attacks among some of the men taking it.

In time, we learned more about the true cause of reduced testosterone. Closer scrutiny revealed that many of the affected men were overweight and their body fat was producing molecules that caused their low numbers. The recommended treatment to improve testosterone levels should be weight loss rather than a drug.

As science advances and we learn more about the complex interactions between weight and cognitive and metabolic health, we can expect other powerful and unexpected associations to emerge. Almost surely, this expanding body of knowledge will reinforce the actionable conclusions we have already reached about the importance of maintaining metabolic health.

Part V

Heart Disease

Chapter 30

Recommendation: reduce your LDL levels to prevent heart disease

Reducing fast carbs is one valuable strategy for reducing metabolic and cardiovascular disease risk. But science now tells us we can do even more than reduce risk. It is no exaggeration to say we may be able to eliminate the vast majority of atherosclerotic heart disease in our lifetime. This remarkable possibility reflects work that has been done over the past fifty years, culminating in new evidence that has emerged much more recently.

Just as fast carbs are an external toxin that causes damage, LDL is an internal toxin that causes damage. It carries fat molecules through our blood; these molecules eventually make their way into the walls of the blood vessels around the heart and initiate an inflammatory process that paves the way for atherosclerosis. LDL-like particles become trapped as they cross the wall of the blood vessels and trigger a complex process that leads to fat deposits that can restrict blood flow. (While we produce other lipid particles as well, LDL accounts for about 90 percent of those that matter to most of us.) Thanks to rigorous, cross-cutting research, we are no longer limited to merely suggesting that high levels of LDL are associated with heart disease, but can instead state confidently that LDL is a *cause* of heart disease.

The lifetime burden of LDL particles in our bodies is a key determinant of our risk profile, along with hypertension and obesity. In the same way that doctors measure the risk of smoking by the number of "pack years" smoked, the risk of developing serious cardiovascular disease correlates with the total amount of LDL that our bodies produce over a lifetime. Just as Americans changed their behavior once they fully understood the risks of smoking, I'm convinced that they will take similar action once they fully grasp the damage that LDL can do.

Lowering LDL has conclusively been proven to reduce the risk of cardiovascular disease, and the lower the better. For every 40 mg/dL reduction in LDL, risk decreases by about 25 percent. The evidence of this correlation is so strong, and the benefits so dramatic, that the question is no longer "Should you lower your LDL levels?" but rather "How low should you go?"

Until recently, the target LDL level for most adults was 100 mg/dL. Today, especially for those who are at higher risk, that target is often 70 or lower. We are now testing the lower limits of LDL to determine if there are health benefits to reducing it even further and whether doing so could present any dangers of its own. Meanwhile, most Americans are far from even the traditional target—people who have been diagnosed as at risk for heart disease often have LDL levels of 112 or more.

Half a century ago, the McGovern Committee recognized that high levels of LDL were associated with atherosclerosis and cardiovascular disease and advised Americans to reduce their intake of saturated fat. They were right. Reducing foods high in saturated fats is important. But what the Senate committee failed to recognize, and what too many scientists still don't emphasize, is the danger of replacing that fat with highly processed carbs.

Chapter 31

LDL causes heart disease

In 2017, two Australian researchers, Peter Clifton and Jennifer Keogh, examined a trove of studies on the connection between LDL and diet. This included new research from two large cohorts: the Nurses' Health Study and the Health Professionals Follow-Up Study. Scientists often return to earlier research and perform what is called *meta-analysis*—that is, they treat the underlying data from several studies as one giant study, thereby increasing the data pool and the accuracy of the findings. This was such an undertaking.

Clifton and Keogh combined data from sixty-seven studies performed over seven years (between 2010 and 2017) and reached an unambiguous conclusion: *reducing saturated fat does not lower the rate of cardiac disease if it is replaced with processed carbohydrates*. Their analysis offers strong evidence that fast carbs pose as much of a threat to cardiac health as saturated fat. They also concluded that replacing saturated fat with poly- or monounsaturated fat (for example, olive oil), along with unprocessed carbohydrates, reduces cardiovascular risk.

While this study caught my attention, it was another set of research that demonstrated to me the profound opportunity we have to markedly reduce the incidence of cardiovascular disease. The data presented at the European Society of Cardiology's meetings in Munich and Paris over the past several years, which were first published in the 2017 issue of the *European Heart Journal* under the unambiguous title "Low-Density Lipoproteins Cause Atherosclerotic Cardiovascular Disease," opened my eyes to the possibility of practically eradicating cardiovascular disease.

Causality—that is, a direct link between one variable and an illness or disease—can be hard to prove. When I was the commissioner of the FDA, we insisted that before drugs were approved for use, they had to undergo large-scale randomized trials. In general, such trials involve dividing subjects randomly into two groups: one group is given the experimental drug, while the other either gets a placebo or the drug that is the current standard of care for the condition of concern.

The object of randomized trials is to isolate one variable, in this case the drug being tested. We want to make sure that if people get better, it can be attributed to the drug and not to some other factor—for example, dietary or metabolic changes, or even unconscious interference by the researchers.

The link between LDL and cardiovascular disease

represents a more complicated case because LDL levels are controlled by so many factors. Our bodies can produce their own lipids, so diet is not the only source of LDL. What makes the *European Heart Journal* paper so compelling is that it offers a naturally occurring randomized trial that isolated LDL as a cause of heart disease. Researchers found patients with genetic mutations that either significantly increased or decreased the level of LDL in their blood. These mutations can be considered truly random, and they affect only one health factor—LDL levels. This allowed the researchers to focus on a single question: What is the effect of such mutations on cardiovascular outcomes?

The authors of the paper looked at over two hundred studies involving more than two million subjects, including people who had one of the naturally occurring mutations. The researchers also looked at clinical trials to see if there was a clear relationship between lipid-lowering drugs and lowered risk of cardiovascular disease.

Their findings were resoundingly clear. There is a "remarkably consistent" association between LDL in the blood and the risk of cardiovascular disease, wrote the researchers. The study "provides overwhelming clinical evidence that LDL [causes atherosclerotic cardiovascular disease] and that lowering LDL reduces the risk of cardiovascular events."

The causal role played by LDL in atherosclerotic heart disease was reinforced in the 2019 guidelines from the European Society of Cardiology and the European Atherosclerosis Society, which again concluded that LDL and other ApoB-containing lipoproteins cause atherosclerotic cardiovascular disease. ApoB is the name that is given to the protein on the surface of these lipid particles in our bloodstream. These ApoB-containing molecules include both LDL and triglyceride particles.

In addition to these findings, randomized clinical drug trials carried out over the past decade have demonstrated unequivocally that the lower the level of LDL, the lower the associated atherosclerotic cardiovascular risk. As Dr. Richard Nesto, who heads the cardiovascular medicine department at the Lahey Hospital in Burlington, Massachusetts, says, "There is absolutely no level of LDL below which you do not additionally benefit by further lowering LDL." This data is not limited to any one class of drugs, such as the statins, which means that the finding is not unique to any of the drugs, but to the LDL particle itself.

I have many well-meaning colleagues who have studied the effects of low-carbohydrate diets despite criticism from the mainstream nutrition community. These individuals deserve enormous credit for long ago recognizing the dangers associated with rapidly absorbable carbohydrates. But their work has one serious shortcoming: it fails to adequately take into account the dangers of saturated fat and its role in elevating LDL.

These shortcomings are not of anyone's making. Rather, they result from the inherent limitations of the type of nutritional epidemiological studies that make it hard to reach reliable conclusions. Unlike these nutrition studies, because of very strict requirements that we imposed at FDA for cardiac drugs, the studies I rely on about the benefits of lowering LDL are based on very large, well-controlled clinical studies.

Chapter 32

———

Eating less starch reduces salt intake and lowers blood pressure

While our focus in this section is on LDL, I want to focus on another core measure that demands our attention: blood pressure, which is one of the most modifiable risk factors we face. Three diseases associated with aging—heart failure, stroke, and dementia—are all linked to blood pressure.

Reduce your blood pressure by nearly 10 millimeters of mercury, in combination with reducing your LDL levels, and you reduce the lifetime risk of cardiovascular disease by at least 80 percent. The risk of cardiovascular death falls by two-thirds.

Losing weight is exceptionally important for lowering blood pressure, which falls between 0.5 and 1.0 mmHg for every pound you lose. Reducing salt intake is also key; more salt in your diet translates to higher blood pressure, especially as we grow older. "If we could impact salt and weight beginning early in life, we can avoid a lot of harm," asserts Dr. Paul Whelton, who was involved in the blood pressure guidelines designed to direct the nation. According to Dr. Michel Burnier, an emeritus professor at University Hospital of Lausanne, Switzerland, "There is increasing evidence regarding the benefits of reducing salt intake to prevent cardiovascular disease even in the absence of powerful randomized controlled trials."

Americans are consuming salt at higher-than-recommended levels, but the medical community has not been paying enough attention to that. In fact, they don't even know how much salt is in their own diet, as Dr. Stephen Devries discovered when he asked a group of cardiologists how much salt they had consumed the previous day. Not one could answer the question.

An easy way to make a difference in this critical health area is to avoid the three processed foods with the highest amounts of salt—commercially produced bread, processed meats, and pizza. Packaged snack foods like chips, pretzels and crackers, and cereals are high-salt products. None of that should be a surprise, because starch itself is so bland that the industry knows these foods are not palatable without salt. In the same way that sugar and fat is added to a starch base to create hyper-palatable processed food items, harmful amounts of salt are often hiding in that unholy mix as well. These additives are used to mask off-notes in processed products.

Dr. Whelton says that from his perspective as a blood pressure clinician, when you get on in age there are three diseases you should worry about—stroke, heart failure, and dementia—all three related to blood pressure. According to the National Academy of Medicine, "35 percent of myocardial infarction and stroke events, 49 percent of heart failure episodes, and 24 percent of premature deaths" are attributed to high blood pressure. "We need to up our game," said Dr. Whelton, by being more aggressive in treating blood pressure. For both weight and salt reduction, the greater the reduction, the more we can lower the risk.

Chapter 33

Diet or medicine to lower LDL?
Probably both

At a 2019 meeting of the European Society of Cardiology in Paris, Dr. Salim Yusuf, the chair of cardiology at McMaster University, suggested that it was time to stop quibbling over saturated fats and other dietary recommendations and intensively treat people with statins, the medications prescribed to inhibit production of LDL in the liver, and with therapies to control blood pressure. His provocative assertion is that medication will have a much bigger impact than "tinkering about with little things that have tiny effects, like salt reduction or arguing about saturated fats." Such a strategy, he contended, would be far better than any nutritional guidelines because we now have drugs that are much more powerful than diet alone.

There is some appeal to this argument because we can indeed reduce LDL and blood pressure dramatically with pharmaceuticals. But my conversations with Dr. Eugene Braunwald, perhaps the most prominent cardiologist in the world and a strong advocate of intensive lipid and blood pressure drug therapy, highlighted the limitations of that singular focus. I asked him if we should forgo dietary preventive measures and just advocate for drug therapy.

Dr. Braunwald resisted the idea—correctly, in my opinion. His reservations did not reflect qualms about safety or possible adverse events from pharmacological therapy (although there are some risks, including the small potential of statins to lead to new-onset diabetes and an uncertain risk of hemorrhagic stroke). It was because he felt strongly that diet was the important first step in prevention, and any recommendation to emphasize pharmacology exclusively could minimize the broader benefits of a healthy diet. While it is critically important to address LDL and blood pressure, treating obesity is every bit as vital in order to prevent diabetes, atherosclerotic cardiovascular disease, and cognitive decline.

Dr. Braunwald emphasized that diet alone may not be enough. And again, he is right. We may be able to eradicate much of heart disease in this generation, but it will likely take a combination of drugs that lower lipid levels and blood pressure *and* diet to accomplish that.

LDL is not only an internal toxin—it is a lifelong toxin. LDL accumulates in heart vessel walls over our entire lifetime. Reducing LDL over a lifetime is more important than short-term reductions, according to Dr. John Kastelein at the University of Amsterdam, a colleague of Dr. Braunwald, as the benefits of reducing LDL are related to the magnitude and duration of that reduction. To prevent atherosclerotic cardiovascular disease, we need to take steps early in life to reduce our LDL levels.

"We are all accumulating atherosclerosis in our arteries in a way that has major future cardiovascular risk," says Dr. John Deanfield of University College London. "Early action for lifetime cardiovascular risk reduction is the key," Dr. Deanfield said. "Modest lowering sustained for many years in blood pressure and blood lipids may have a profound effect."

Chapter 34

Recommendation:
engage in daily moderate-intensity exercise to stay healthy

Almost everyone will agree on the importance of getting regular exercise, but too many of us don't follow that simple recommendation. Along with cultivating a lifelong practice of avoiding fast carbs, a lifelong practice of regular exercise is one of the baseline strategies for maintaining a healthy weight and lowering your risk of developing metabolic and cardiovascular disease.

As with diet, there are a lot of competing exercise regimens and recommendations that offer various and sometimes conflicting advice. My recommendation is straightforward: everyone should aim to exercise five days a week, for a minimum of thirty to sixty minutes, with an eye toward a weekly total of at least 150 minutes and preferably closer to 300 minutes. You can do this at a moderate level of intensity, or exercise more vigorously and gain the same benefit in perhaps half the time. Most of your activity should be aerobic, but strengthening the muscles through some form of resistance training at least twice a week is also important.

Jim Hill, a professor at the University of Alabama at Birmingham, says there are two reasons physical activity is so crucial. "First, it increases your energy expenditure and allows you to eat more," he explained. Without exercise, people who lose weight have to sustain the caloric restrictions that got them there, despite a hormonal response that cries out for more food. The body compensates for reduced intake by lowering its resting metabolic rate, using less energy, and storing more fat. That process creates what Hill calls an energy gap that is hard for almost anyone to overcome.

"The more you try to [fill this gap] with food restriction alone, the more likely you are to fail. Some people can do it, but most people need to use exercise to fill at least part of this gap," he said.

Second, exercise helps to regulate metabolism. Over the course of the day, there are generally periods when we eat fat, carbohydrates, or protein, and others when we are eating nothing at all. If you are healthy, your metabolic system adjusts easily, keeping caloric intake and physiological activity in tandem, and body weight remains stable. But if your metabolism is out of balance, then the body responds by slowing metabolism even as caloric intake increases.

Exercise, Hill said, can "fix your broken metabolism."

He later added, "Physical activity is the major predictor of metabolic flexibility and inflexibility."

This is clear when we look at the problem of insulin resistance. When insulin acts on glucose, 80 percent of that glucose is taken up by the muscles; the liver, fat tissue, and brain tissue dispose of the rest. In a prediabetic or diabetic state, the efficiency of those processes is undermined. Glucose uptake by skeletal muscles and other tissue is insufficient, and the sugars continue to circulate in the bloodstream with rising blood glucose levels.

Because muscles are the dominant storehouse for glucose, many researchers believe that their resistance to insulin is the primary defect that allows prediabetes and diabetes to develop. Jacob Haus of the University of Michigan says that exercise helps the muscles to take up more glucose from the bloodstream and metabolize it. Exercise also helps to increase insulin sensitivity in fatty tissue and the liver, enabling those depots to dispose of glucose more efficiently as well.

In one study, Haus compared three groups to determine the influence of exercise on insulin sensitivity—healthy individuals; those with some degree of impaired sensitivity to insulin; and people with diabetes. After three months of aerobic exercise, sixty minutes a day, five days a week, at 75 percent of the body's maximum oxygen intake capacity and 80 to 85 percent of its maximum heart rate, the investigators recorded improvements in all three populations.

It doesn't even have to take that long to see results. Haus and his team also found that seven consecutive days of aerobic exercise raised insulin sensitivity by 45 percent, leading to more glucose uptake by the muscles and increased glucose metabolism.

How do we translate the science into an exercise regimen that works? First, keep in mind that moderately intense physical activity means different things to different people, and depends on your baseline level of fitness. Doctors and nutritionists have various ways of measuring exercise intensity. For example, they can assess how close you are to your body's maximum capacity to absorb oxygen (VO_2 max). But that's not something you can do on your own. What you can do instead is establish an appropriate target heart rate, with guidance from your doctor, and then wear one of the many types of monitors available to help you measure it. With moderately intense activity, such as brisk walking, doubles tennis, recreational biking, or swimming, you can reach 50 to 70 percent of the heart's maximum capacity. More vigorous exercise uses up more energy—running a ten-minute mile, for example, can raise your heart rate to 70 to 85 percent of maximum capacity.

Your own perception of how hard you are working is also a reasonable measure—if you are breathing hard, but can still carry on a conversation and are perspiring lightly after about ten minutes, your exercise is probably moderately intense. In a vigorous workout, you should be breathing too hard to talk much and perspiring within a few minutes after initiating exercise.

The good news is that if you are significantly overweight,

or are new to exercise, the benefits accrue very quickly. But individuals with prediabetes or full-blown disease will find that they have to do more to get the same clinical benefit as someone who is metabolically healthy. The more dysfunctional your metabolism is when you start, the longer you will have to work to see the benefits. But exercise at any point, from any fitness baseline, will lead to results. In other words, it's never too late.

Walk a little farther, or more often; climb a flight of stairs instead of taking the elevator; you can reduce your glycemic load somewhat beginning on the very first day you exercise. The effect of multiple activities is cumulative, and consistency is critical. "You're only as good as your last exercise," says Haus, emphasizing the importance of an ongoing commitment.

Frequency, intensity, duration, and type of activity all influence the effects of exercise, but the bottom line is that the relationship between cardiorespiratory fitness and insulin sensitivity is powerful and protective. Being fit allows you to take in more oxygen when you exercise, which increases your endurance and makes you more sensitive to insulin. Over time, sustained moderate-intensity physical activity—not once, but day after day for a lifetime—is essential for weight maintenance, metabolic control, and cardiovascular health.

———

Part VI

The Optimal Diet

Chapter 35

———

Most successful diets have one thing in common: limited fast carbs

I understand all too well that those of us who have been engaged in a lifelong struggle with weight are exhausted from confusing and often contradictory recommendations about what to eat. Avoid saturated fat and you can wind up eating too many fast carbs. Avoid carbs and you can wind up eating too much saturated fat.

What, then, should we eat? Fortunately, there is a realistic and practical answer to that question, and it is quite simple. A truly healthy diet—one that allows us to achieve and maintain a healthy weight while helping to prevent metabolic disorders and cardiovascular disease—looks something like this:

1. **Reduce or eliminate consumption of processed carbs.**

2. **Eat minimal saturated fat.**

3. Eat slow carbs that are high in fiber and nutrients.

I am not endorsing a specific diet plan, but rather an approach to eating that considers all of our needs. Remarkably, there is some core agreement about these recommendations in the sometimes rancorous, often competitive nutrition and weight communities.

That became apparent to me at a session of the American Heart Association conference titled "Diets from Vegan to Ketogenic: What's the Best for Cardiovascular Health and for Which Patient?" Speaker after speaker presented their data supporting a particular diet—Mediterranean, plant-based, high protein, ketogenic. Though polite, each speaker clearly wanted to convince the audience that his or her dietary vision was the one true path to health.

First to speak was Dr. Sarah Hallberg, medical director at Virta Health, a startup that creates products to treat type 2 diabetes. She was an advocate for a ketogenic diet, which is extremely low in carbs (including slow carbs). By denying the body glucose, ketogenic diets aim to force the body to burn ketones and fat.

Dr. Hallberg was determined to disabuse the audience of the notion that keto was "the hot-dog-and-cheese diet," insisting that it can be a nutritional plan based on whole foods. A diet low in carbohydrates needn't overemphasize protein, she said. The cornerstone of Hallberg's version of keto is fat, but she promotes monounsaturated fatty acids, stressing the importance of olive oil to her patients. She also recommends using monounsaturated fats and avoiding highly refined and processed vegetable oils.

Dr. Hallberg explained that, unlike the extreme low-carb diets of the 1990s, a modern keto diet does not prescribe avoiding all carbohydrates. Rather, keto diets emphasize the *source* of carbs—nonstarchy vegetables rather than grains and potatoes. Indeed, Dr. Hallberg recommends that her patients eat five servings of nonstarchy vegetables a day. The diet can also accommodate dairy, nuts and seeds, and some fruit, "especially once people have reversed their metabolic issues," she said. Only grains (including whole grains), potatoes, and sugar remain forbidden.

Next, Dr. Miguel A. Martínez-González, an internationally renowned epidemiologist, presented on the Mediterranean diet, which first earned its name in the 1960s, from Ancel Keys's study of local dietary patterns. "What *is* the Mediterranean diet?" he asked, and then followed up with another question: "Or better, we should say, what is *not* the Mediterranean diet?" He went on to say that not all foods eaten today in Mediterranean countries fit within the confines of the traditional heart-healthy diet. While there are multiple nutritional patterns in the region, most time-honored regimens put olive oil at the center of the diet, while also emphasizing fish, nuts and legumes, fruit, and vegetables. And, Dr. González was quick to add, wine—preferably red, and always in moderation.

Slight differences in branding notwithstanding, the dueling diets began to seem quite similar, especially with their emphasis on consuming olive oil and avoiding starchy foods.

The third speaker was Dr. Kim Williams, who presented on plant-based diets. His opening salvo was a warning on the hazards of red meat, but he also pointed out that not every vegetarian diet is equally healthy and shared evidence that even vegan diets can be perilous. A vegan who consumes large amounts of juices, refined grains, fried foods, and sweets might be in worse shape, metabolically speaking, than a meat eater: "Drumroll," he proclaimed to underscore his counterintuitive point. "You'd be better off with the bacon."

Again, the dietary recommendations seemed to be inching closer together.

Recognizing a common thread, I decided to act as a peacemaker. At the end of the presentations I went to the microphone.

"Perhaps I can get some agreement. Let me give you a general principle and ask what you think from a public health perspective. Should everyone reduce their consumption of rapidly digestible carbohydrates?"

Initially hesitant, all three speakers nodded their heads.

"Would anyone disagree?" I asked.

Dr. Christopher Gardner from Stanford answered for all: "This group is with you."

Curiously, Dr. Gardner had a similar experience some years before we met at this conference. He, too, had listened to three experts bicker over the exact shape of the ideal diet on a panel he was moderating. Looking for points of agreement, he asked the group whether two basic nutritional tenets were consistent with the food plans each was advocating: eliminating added sugar and refined grains, and replacing most of those foods with vegetables. Once again, there was a consensus.

Gardner's own research also supported that finding. In a study that compared low-carb and low-fat diets, he found that the two groups who were counseled to follow these protocols had lost the same amount of weight, on average. Despite their differences, the meal plans both eliminated sugar and refined grains, while encouraging participants to eat as many vegetables as they could. "We called them 'healthy low-carb' and 'healthy low-fat' diets," he explained.

Gardner lamented to me that health professionals have failed to communicate this coherent and straightforward nutritional advice to the public. "People are confused," he said, distracted by conversations over such seemingly arcane terms as "soluble" and "insoluble" fiber and the "omega-6-to-3 ratio."

Amid a glut of buzzwords, there is solid science behind the imperative to significantly reduce processed carbohydrates—and, fortunately, it's the right approach for all three issues we've been exploring: controlling weight, protecting your metabolic health, and lowering your risk of cardiovascular disease.

Chapter 36

———

A diet emphasizing plants and slow carbs is optimal for your health

As we have seen, it is possible to meet your personal weight goals and maintain good health with many diet programs. Each one presents different challenges and possibilities, and your choice will depend largely on your food preferences and lifestyle. But whether you choose to follow a formal program or not, the path to better health and disease prevention rests on these basic guidelines: reduce or eliminate fast carbs, limit saturated fat (typically found in animal products), and eat plenty of slow carbs like nonstarchy vegetables, whole grains, and fruit.

That said, there is compelling evidence that following a plant-based diet—reducing your consumption of animal products or eliminating them entirely—offers tremendous benefits. One of the most vocal proponents of plant-based eating is Dr. Robert Ostfeld, a Harvard-trained cardiologist. He shared evidence that suggests that a plant-based diet lowers LDL in randomized controlled data as effectively as certain statins. It also lowers C-reactive protein (CRP), a marker of inflammation and cardiovascular risk. In addition, plant-based diets have been shown to lower blood pressure and significantly reduce lipoprotein(a), which is another lipid.

Plant-based diets also improve metabolic health in patients with diabetes. In a randomized control trial of about one hundred people, those on a vegan diet were able to stop taking more diabetes medications than those who followed the recommendations of the American Diabetes Association. The vegans saw greater reductions in their A1c levels (a marker for blood sugar), lost more weight, and lowered their LDL more dramatically.

Dr. Ostfeld pointed to a large-scale study conducted by Dr. Ambika Satija, a postdoctoral fellow in nutrition at Harvard. It demonstrated that the more servings of whole, plant-based foods participants ate, the lower their risk of coronary heart disease. Animal products, including chicken and fish, had the opposite effect (see graph).

"There's similar data for diabetes," Ostfeld pointed out. In a meta-analysis of more than 800,000 people, each daily serving of fruit and vegetables they ate was associated with a 5 percent reduction in mortality risk. In one study looking at the effects of giving up all animal products, the closer participants came to full vegetarianism, the better they did, "in a dose-dependent way," he added. Participants who ate the most plant-based foods had 41 percent lower mortality than those who ate the least.

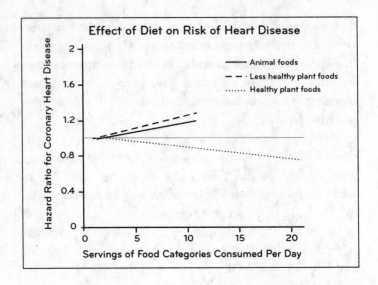

Two caveats: First, this is an observational study, not a controlled trial. Second, just because a food carries the label "plant-based" does not mean that it is a healthy choice. Increasingly, food products are being marketed as plant-based to suggest they are healthier alternatives to meat, dairy, or eggs. But in fact, some of these processed foods contain as much as or more saturated fat than their animal-derived counterparts. For example, Impossible Burger plant-based patties contain 40 percent saturated fat; Beyond Burger contains 30 percent saturated fat. These vegetarian burgers offer as much as or more saturated fat than a similar-size ground beef burger. While they may have an important role in reducing the greenhouse gas emissions associated with meat production, the best plant-based eating style is one that is based primarily on whole foods, not processed meat substitutes.

Whether or not you decide to go fully vegan or vegetarian, the takeaway here is this: plant-based foods deserve a foundational place in your diet.

Chapter 37

The pros and cons of low-carb diets

L ow-carb diets have attracted a significant following in recent years, and there is no doubt that these programs can be effective if sustained over the long term. The amount of carbohydrate restriction on "low carb" varies, from the scant 20 to 50 grams per day prescribed by ketogenic diets that aim to maintain nutritional "ketosis" to more moderate approaches that restrict carbs to 100 to 150 grams per day. The foods that are permissible on these diets also vary. Paleo diets, for example, are a low-carb regimen that emphasizes unprocessed meat, fish, leafy and cruciferous vegetables, eggs, fruit, and nuts. In general, they exclude whole grains (including rice and oats), potatoes, beans and legumes, and dairy products. In a ketogenic diet, permissible carbs come primarily from non-starchy vegetables and, unlike the Paleo Diet, it includes full-fat dairy products such as cheese and cream. But one common thread among all of these protocols is that the majority of calories come from fat.

We've already reviewed the evidence that low-carb diets can lead to dramatic improvements in diabetes. In some of these studies, daily calories were severely limited. But even when food intake was not restricted, the results are remarkable. In one study, subjects on a standard American diet ate about 3,100 calories, but when they switched to a low-carb diet with no caloric restrictions, they ate 1,000 fewer calories a day *on their own*. The resulting effects on glucose control, insulin sensitivity, and daily medication needs were also quite dramatic—in just two weeks there was a 75 percent improvement in insulin sensitivity. In another recent study, this one conducted by Virta Health, Dr. Sarah Hallberg and colleagues found that 74 percent of people with diabetes on a low-carb diet maintained their diet after two years and sustained an average weight loss of nearly thirty pounds. Fifty-three percent of participants had reversed their diabetes.

Despite these benefits, there is legitimate concern from some in the nutrition and medical communities about low-carbohydrate diets that emphasize animal protein and fat over plant-based whole foods. This is especially true for some of the early versions of low-carb diets, such as the one advocated by Dr. Robert Atkins. His red-meat-and-butter approach was not simply low in carbohydrates; it was, by design, high in saturated fat. Premised on the idea that fat (ketones), rather than glucose, is a preferred fuel source, saturated fat is the cornerstone of the Atkins Diet.

As researchers have become increasingly critical of the low-carb community's embrace of saturated fat—which can increase LDL—more recent low-carb diets have attempted to correct for this problem. The recommended revised protocol, said Dr. Amy Goss of the University of Alabama at Birmingham, "is predominantly comprised of whole foods. The fats come from both plant and animal sources: avocado, olive oil, cheese, eggs, salad dressing, salmon, and Greek yogurt." Registered dietitian Dr. Brittanie Volk endorses this whole foods approach to low-carb eating. "Remember, the goal is to gain control of blood sugar, so reducing carbohydrates is a way to achieve such control, which then leads to control over hunger and cravings. When you empower patients to eat in such a way that reduces their hunger and cravings, they can be empowered to make the best nutrition choices."

Yet even these more enlightened diets can raise LDL. Dr. Stephen Phinney, a strong advocate of low-carb eating, cofounded Virta Health, a startup that treats type 2 diabetics with a low-carb diet. He acknowledged concerns about which foods are used as substitutes for carbs and how they impact LDL. In Dr. Hallberg's study, the average increase in LDL was 10 percent after participants switched to a low-carb diet, but a significant number of patients saw their LDL go up by as much as 30 percent.

Dr. Phinney and other proponents of low-carb diets believe such a protocol nonetheless has a positive impact on many other cardiovascular risk factors. He points out, correctly, that lowering weight is by itself highly beneficial, as is lowering triglycerides, blood pressure, and inflammation.

He goes on to argue, as other scientists do, that it is the size of LDL particles that contributes to plaques, not their absolute number. In this theory, bigger LDL particles are thought to be less damaging because of their increased buoyancy and lower risk of getting into the vessel walls. But recent research suggests that it is not the size of LDL particles that most contributes to atherosclerosis and heart disease, but rather the *number* of them, which we can count with the biomarker ApoB protein. The amount of ApoB in your blood best predicts your coronary risk. Triglycerides, as well as LDL, increase the quantity of ApoB-containing particles, but eating fewer carbs and losing weight drives that number down. Saturated fat generally maintains or increases ApoB levels and the number of LDL particles.

A growing number of cardiac scientists agree. "The most well-established risk factor for cardiovascular disease is LDL," Dr. Manuel Mayr, an eminent molecular cardiologist at King's College London, told me. "It would be difficult to argue that a treatment that increases LDL reduces cardiovascular risk." Mayr does not feel that other positive metabolic and cardiovascular benefits could offset the dangers of raising LDL.

Dr. Brian Ference, a cardiologist and genetic epidemiologist at the University of Cambridge, agrees with this conclusion, commenting, "My own view is that, on a population scale, we can't recommend saturated fats because in general we know that they will, on average, increase LDL."

All of these findings point to the necessity of being

mindful about what to eat when we replace carbs in a low-carb diet. Our primary goal should be to reduce LDL as much as possible, especially among those of us who are at risk for cardiovascular disease (and as we age, that group includes more and more of us). Dr. Jeannie Tay at the University of Alabama at Birmingham showed in a clinical trial that a diet that emphasized nuts and vegetables, and was low in both carbs and saturated fat, reduced spikes in blood glucose and the need for diabetes medication without raising LDL. Even people who are already on lipid-lowering drugs can further lower their LDL levels modestly by moving from saturated to unsaturated fats.

One caveat: there are overwhelming data from clinical trials that demonstrate that lowering LDL by drugs has a marked effect on reduction of cardiovascular disease. Unlike that data, there are not equivalent modern day clinical trials that demonstrate cardiovascular benefit when LDL is lowered by diet. Such a result is, however, a fair extrapolation based on all the evidence.

Chapter 38

———

Don't consume processed meats

Though we should aim to eat more plants, it's unlikely that everyone will choose to become vegetarian or vegan. But there is one type of animal product that we can agree to moderate our intake of, if not forgo: processed meats.

The World Health Organization defines processed meat as "meat that has been transformed through salting, curing, fermentation, smoking or other processes to enhance flavor or improve preservation. Most processed meats contain pork or beef, but processed meats may also contain other red meats, poultry, offal, or meat by-products such as blood. Examples of processed meat include hot dogs (frankfurters), ham, sausages, corned beef, and biltong or beef jerky as well as canned meat and meat-based preparations and sauces."

Slightly less off-putting, if only because it's less detailed, is the definition of the American Institute for Cancer Research: "meat preserved by smoking, curing, or salting, or addition of chemical preservatives."

Processed meat is classified as a category 1 carcinogen by the World Health Organization, in the same category as tobacco smoking or asbestos exposure (but the WHO has made clear that that does not mean they are equally dangerous). The International Agency for Research on Cancer has calculated that "each 50-gram portion [a small hot dog] of processed meat eaten daily increases the risk of colorectal cancer by 18 percent." Moreover, according to the Global Burden of Disease project, "about 34,000 cancer deaths worldwide per year are attributable to diets high in processed meat."

If that's not enough to warn you off of the stuff, coronary heart disease and stroke are also associated with processed meats. "If everybody went from processed red meat to just regular red meat, we would dramatically decrease cardiovascular death in this country," said Dr. Kim Williams, the former president of the American College of Cardiology. Williams, a vegan who nonetheless understands why people enjoy red meat, added, "Every time you are able to replace animal protein with plant protein, you get this amount of decrease in mortality. The worst, by far, is processed red meat."

Here are the labels for two common processed red-meat products:

Hillshire Farm Hot Links: 100% Premium Pork. No Fillers. No MSG Added. Ingredients: pork, water, contains 2% or less: corn syrup, salt, potassium lactate, flavoring, brown sugar, dextrose, spices (including hot red pepper, ground red pepper, and capsicum), pork stock, sodium phosphate, sodium diacetate, sodium erythorbate, sunflower oil, sodium nitrite. Made with beef collagen casing.

Boar's Head Bologna: 0g Trans fat per serving. Good source of protein. Gluten free. Milk free. No MSG. Ingredients: Pork, water, beef, salt. Less than 1.5% of dextrose, sugar, sodium phosphate, paprika, sodium erythorbate, flavorings, sodium nitrite.

Two large studies address the effects of this panoply of additives and preservatives.

A 2010 meta-analysis reviewed studies that included 1.2 million people from the United States, Europe, Asia, and Australia. The report concluded that the sodium levels and nitrate preservatives in processed meats could be linked to a higher risk of cardiovascular disease and type 2 diabetes mellitus. "Dietary sodium significantly increases blood pressure, and habitual consumption may also worsen arterial compliance [responsiveness] and promote vascular stiffness. Nitrates and their byproducts experimentally promote atherosclerosis and vascular dysfunction, reduce insulin secretion, and impair glucose tolerance."

The researchers concluded that each daily serving of processed meat was associated with a 42 percent higher risk of cardiovascular heart disease and a 19 percent higher risk of type 2 diabetes mellitus.

A 2016 review of the twenty-year Nurses' Health Study

found increased mortality associated with consumption of processed red meats from all causes, not just cancer or cardiovascular disease. The review went on to state, "Moreover, we observed that substitution of plant protein for animal protein from a variety of food sources, particularly processed red meat, was associated with a lower risk of mortality."

In a study of this size, the health of participants varied widely. There were smokers, heavy drinkers, people who never exercised, people who exercised daily, and everyone in between. The researchers observed, "Those with unhealthy lifestyles consumed more processed and unprocessed red meat, whereas the healthy-lifestyle group consumed more fish and chicken as animal protein sources, suggesting that different protein sources, at least partly, contributed to the observed variation. . . . Red meat, especially processed red meat, showed a much stronger [risk of death] than fish and poultry."

In a recent and highly controversial set of five studies published in *Annals of Internal Medicine* and reported on the front page of the *New York Times*, researchers concluded that the benefits of lessening red meat consumption (a reduction of one to six heart attacks per thousand, or seven fewer cancer deaths per thousand) was not significant enough, in their opinion, to justify curtailing meat intake. This conclusion was made despite the fact that the analyses found a statistically significant association between less consumption of processed and red meat and less cardiac disease, cancer, diabetes, and deaths from any cause—a finding that is consistent with many previous studies.

It's important to understand why this study, and its conclusions, are flawed. In any nutritional epidemiological study that aims to assess the danger posed by a particular food, one must take into consideration the control against which the food in question is being compared. In this case, any accurate assessment of whether or not meat is harmful must weigh the risk of consuming meat against the risk of consuming an alternative source of nutrition. Compared to a standard American diet comprising fast carbs, eating meat isn't going to demonstrate any worse outcomes. Compared to a high-quality plant-based diet, however, the data would most likely indicate that eating meat is associated with higher LDL than with a plant-based protocol.

As the media coverage of this study—and the ensuing outrage it generated—reveals, reporting on nutrition often leaves people confused about how best to eat for their health. Unfortunately, that confusion obscures the simple fact we do know: that lowering LDL will markedly reduce our risk of cardiovascular disease, and lowering LDL begins with what we choose to eat.

Chapter 39

Your diet doesn't have to be perfect

Consider two environments: one is abundant with highly palatable processed foods, including fast carbs; the other offers only whole foods and no fast carbs. Our weight will settle at two very different points depending on which of these environments we spend time in. In my own experience, I always used to lose weight when I went away to summer camp—where I was physically active and didn't have the option of eating junk food all day long, and where the cues that triggered my overeating were absent. When I returned home at the end of the summer, I would gain it all back again. To this day, when I travel to certain parts of the world where the food environment is very different from ours in the U.S., I come back with fewer pounds on my frame. These environments stand out for me because they are places where I have lost weight without much struggle or effort. I was able to eat comfortably while my weight adjusted to a new "settling point."

Of course, we have little control over the food environment outside our homes. The rules governing food labeling, marketing, and processing are set by government policy, and the products on store shelves reflect consumer demand and industry marketing. I hope we can achieve change in all of these realms, but meanwhile, there are simple things each of us can do to exert a little more control over our individual food environments.

Eating is at once a conscious and unconscious behavior. Thoughts flow into your consciousness, often triggered by sights, smells, locations, or bodily sensations, and you begin to act. Your hand moves toward a plate of cookies; you walk to the refrigerator; you may even begin eating automatically, without deliberate intention. At some point, it seems that your attention has been hijacked. An internal dialogue may ensue, marked by intrusive thoughts: *I really should stop.* When you attempt to abstain from a particular food, cravings result, which often leads to overeating or bingeing on the very food you are trying to avoid.

One of the goals of any weight-loss plan must be to stem this rising tide long before it reaches your conscious awareness. To control what is unconscious, you'll need to understand what is happening in your body and recognize that although part of your brain is telling you to eat those chips, you don't really want to do so, because you know they are literally killing you. If you think, "I want it, but I can't have it," then you will obsess about it and feel deprived. But if you think, "I don't want that, it is poison to me," the struggle becomes easier. Notice I didn't say "easy": just "easier."

One of the traps of overeating is that you can become preoccupied by what you perceive as your failure. When the reward circuits of your brain overcome your conscious desire not to eat, you inevitably feel terrible about your behavior. And, of course, people often react to the resulting stress with the completely counterproductive response of eating.

That's why I encourage you to be forgiving with yourself. Try to let go of the guilt or shame if—when—you don't follow your own rules. This is not to say you shouldn't care. You should care deeply about getting healthy and staying healthy. But it's important to acknowledge that this is hard work, and it is a learning process.

I no longer feel trapped in my own body, nor do I feel that my eating is out of control. Gone are the constant ruminations—*I shouldn't eat that . . . Well, maybe a little . . . No, I really shouldn't.* Well, in truth, they are perhaps not completely gone, but they have quieted enough to allow me to substitute another thought: "I don't really want that; it is killing me."

It's not that I am invulnerable to the instant gratifications of processed carbohydrates. Food cues remain salient; this fact is part of our biological hardwiring. But the fixation is muted, more easily brushed aside. Having learned that eating fast carbs and other processed foods results in no enduring reward, my response to them has gradually become less automatic. And with my metabolism in a healthier state, my biology no longer stimulates overeating.

I freely admit that I don't always follow my own recommendations. Sugar, in particular, has proven especially challenging to eliminate. But I don't necessarily need to earn an A for my accomplishments here. I am a B student, still striving, and for now, that's the best I can do. And that's okay.

In the Public Interest:
Changing Our Food Environment

The industry culpability in promoting fast carbs emerges clearly in this story. But I tried to give companies the benefit of the doubt when I asked a spokesperson at General Mills about the effects of its products. Surely, I suggested, the industry had considered the weight and metabolic challenges most people face and recognized that consumers should be markedly reducing their consumption of rapidly absorbable glucose. Hadn't they?

My wishful thinking was revealed when the company responded to my queries with the claim that "overall, food patterns and dietary habits are more relevant to maintaining healthy blood glucose levels, rather than any single food." To me, that was another way of saying, "We aren't responsible for what you eat, even though we flood the supermarket shelves with excess amounts of rapidly absorbable starches."

The reality is that these enormous companies can only

defend their products if they are going to survive. It's just not possible to make the same profits by selling broccoli, strawberries, and rolled oats. They are going to keep urging us to eat their processed foods until they are forced to change by public demand and government action. What can be done?

First, education. We have to make all Americans aware of the dangers of rapidly absorbable predigested starch and its omnipresence in our food chain. That awareness will spur consumer and voter demand for new products.

Second, government action. The dietary guidelines designed to help consumers make healthy choices must change. We should establish a National Institute of Nutrition to study this issue, conduct rigorous research, and create accurate, easy-to-understand recommendations that cut through often contradictory and confusing arguments. The federal government spends a woefully inadequate sum on nutrition research, especially by contrast with national spending on candy purchases, which is about $40 billion per year.

Can these measures produce a massive shift in our eating habits? It's a tall order, and it's important to note the socioeconomic factors involved in such a shift. Right now, it is more expensive to eat healthy unprocessed foods than processed starch-heavy foods. Those with discretionary income will be able to change their patterns more easily; those with limited means face an even greater challenge. What can government do to help *all* Americans? What industry regulations are needed to force this change? These are urgent questions that demand comprehensive answers and decisive action.

The choices we need to make as individuals to achieve better health are clear, but the path to national health policies still needs to be mapped. Without doubt, to improve and save lives, we need to chart that path now.

Meal Charts

Fast Carbs, Slow Carbs, Low Carbs

I challenged Dr. Nicola Guess, a registered dietitian with a PhD in nutrition who is a research fellow at King's College London and an associate professor at the University of Westminster, to create menus that show examples of fast-carb, slow-carb, and low-carb meal plans. The objective is to move away from a fast-carb diet. For people who struggle with their weight, both a slow-carb and a low-carb diet are shown in recognition that people will need to determine their own optimal places on the continuum between slow carb and low carb. I then engaged in a dialogue with Nicola to discuss the thinking behind the menus. Our question-and-answer session follows the menus.

Monday

	FAST CARBS	SLOW CARBS	LOW CARBS
Breakfast	Blueberry Cheerios (A) Coffee, sugar, milk	Steel-cut oats (B), blueberries Coffee, non-sugar sweetener	Greek yogurt (C), sliced almonds, and blueberries Coffee, non-sugar sweetener (D)
Lunch	Flour tortilla with beef and cheese, salad	Blue corn tortilla (E) with beef and cheese, salad	Beef, cheese, and avocado (F) over a bed of fresh greens
Dinner	Chicken breast with a large serving of short-grain white rice*	Chicken breast with lentils and a small serving of basmati rice* (G)	Chicken and roasted vegetables (H)

(A) Most commercially packaged cereals are high in sugar, with some form of sugar (brown rice syrup, etc.) listed as one of the first ingredients on the label. Replace boxed cereals with whole, sugar-free cereal grains like oats and add whole natural fruit to taste.

(B) Steel-cut oats are a great choice as they are an intact grain and contain no sugar. In contrast, instant oatmeal is made from processed oats and contains added sugars.

---

* Choose a healthy sauce or dressing to your taste, e.g., pesto, tahini, or a simple lemon dressing with fresh herbs.

(C) By removing the oats you remove most of the carbs. Yogurt contains a small amount of natural carbohydrate in the form of lactose, but only about eight grams per six ounces. Topping with almonds and blueberries will add protein and fiber to help keep you full.

(D) Ideally, coffee should be consumed without any added sugars, but if you prefer a sweeter taste, a non-sugar sweetener is preferable to sugar.

(E) Tortillas made from corn, and in particular blue corn, contain more slow carbs than a flour tortilla, which is the definition of a fast carb.

(F) Removing the tortilla eliminates most of the carbs in this meal. By adding avocado, you add healthy fat and help ensure you don't feel deprived. (Although avocado is 10 percent carb by weight, note that the vast majority of this is fiber and will not cause an increase in blood sugar.)

(G) Short-grain white rice is a fast carb. Basmati rice is slower, but you can help slow down the absorption even more by replacing some of the basmati rice with lentils, which are high in fiber and protein.

(H) By removing the rice, you are left with very few carbs. Roast high-fiber cruciferous vegetables like cauliflower, Brussels sprouts, and broccoli in a healthy fat like olive oil to complete the meal.

Tuesday

	FAST CARBS	SLOW CARBS	LOW CARBS
Breakfast	White bread toast, butter, jelly Orange juice	Pumpernickel bread* (A), cream cheese, and smoked salmon	Soft-boiled eggs with avocado and smoked salmon (B)
Lunch	Tuna and mayonnaise on white bread	Cold tuna and pasta salad (C)	Tuna and green salad with almonds and olives (D)
Dinner	Pan-fried fish, vegetables, and rice	Pan-fried fish, vegetables, and tabbouleh† (E)	Pan-fried fish, extra vegetables drizzled generously with olive oil (F)

(A) White bread plus jelly is a double whammy of fast carbs. In contrast, the carbs in traditional pumpernickel bread, not the kind made with white flour, are slow, and cream cheese and salmon add healthy dairy fats and protein, which help slow down absorption even more.

---

* Sometimes rye bread or pumpernickel bread are terms used interchangeably. For both products, look for "coarsely-ground rye berries/kernels" or "whole rye berries/kernels" on the label and avoid those that contain wheat flour.

† Tabbouleh is a Mediterranean dish made with chopped parsley, mint, onions, lemon juice, and bulgur wheat.

(B) By removing the bread you remove most of the carbs. Eggs add protein and avocados are a source of healthy fats to help keep you full.

(C) The carbohydrate in cooled pasta is more resistant to digestion, which makes the carbohydrate release more slowly into the bloodstream.

(D) By removing the pasta, you cut the carbs. Adding healthy fat sources like almonds to your green salad will help keep you full and provide additional essential nutrients.

(E) Instead of rice, which is a fast carb, serve tabbouleh as an accompaniment. The intact grain in bulgur wheat makes it a slow carb.

(F) By removing the tabbouleh, you remove most of the carbs. Add extra vegetables and olive oil for satiating fiber and fat.

Wednesday

	FAST CARBS	SLOW CARBS	LOW CARBS
Breakfast	Flavored low-fat yogurt, granola bar	Plain Greek yogurt (A) Sprinkle of whole oats, handful of pecans, and sliced banana (B)	Plain Greek yogurt Handful of pecans and raspberries (C)
Lunch	Bagel with cream cheese and side salad	Falafel with hummus and side salad (D)	Chicken breast, hummus, and side salad (E)
Dinner	Grilled fish with fries and side salad	Grilled fish with lentil salad (F)	Grilled fish and salad with added pumpkin seeds and pine nuts (G)

(A) Yogurts are often full of added sugars—some contain as much as three teaspoons of sugar per serving. Always choose plain yogurt instead of flavored varieties, and select Greek whenever possible for extra protein.

(B) Beware of granolas, even those marketed as healthy—they often use processed grains and a lot of added sugars. You can make your own granola with oats, nuts, and seeds, or just add some intact oats (such as steel-cut oats), pecans, and sliced banana to the yogurt instead.

(C) By removing the oats, you remove most of the carbs. Depending on your desired carb limit, replacing banana with low-sugar, high-fiber strawberries or raspberries can lower the carb content by more than ten grams.

(D) A bagel made with processed wheat flour is the definition of a fast carb. Falafel is made with chickpeas, which offer protein and is a slower carb.

(E) By having chicken breast instead of falafel, you remove most of the carbs. The hummus and a side salad of mixed leafy greens ensure the meal is fiber- and nutrient-rich.

(F) Fries are both high fat and a fast carb—a combination that tends to drive overconsumption. Ditch the starches and serve the fish with slow carbs in the form of lentils.

(G) Removing the lentils removes most of the carbs. Adding a handful of pumpkin seeds and pine nuts reduces the amount of carb. (Although pumpkin seeds seem to have a lot of carbs in them, per the label, the vast majority of this is completely indigestible fiber.)

Thursday

	FAST CARBS	SLOW CARBS	LOW CARBS
Breakfast	Soft-boiled or scrambled egg, hash browns Orange juice	Soft-boiled or scrambled egg, slice of toasted grain bread (A) Whole orange cut in quarters (B)	Soft-boiled or scrambled egg, smoked salmon and spinach (C) Handful of strawberries (D)
Lunch	Instant noodles	Stir fry with zucchini noodles (E) and vegetables	Beef strips and vegetable stir fry (F)
Dinner	Steak with mashed potatoes and gravy	Beef with noodles and root vegetables (e.g., sweet potato) (G)	Beef with root vegetables (e.g., sweet potato) (H)

(A) Hash browns are processed fast carbs that are also high fat. Choose a small amount of toasted whole grain bread to accompany the egg instead.

(B) Juice lacks the fiber of the fruit's flesh to help slow digestion and prevent insulin spikes. Select the whole fruit instead.

(C) By removing the bread, you remove most of the carbs. Adding smoked salmon and some spinach (or other leafy vegetable) adds nutrients and healthy fats and helps you feel full.

(D) Depending on your desired carb limit, replacing a whole orange with strawberries can lower the carb content by about seven to ten grams.

(E) Rice noodles are a fast carb. Instead choose zucchini noodles, which are a slower carb, and add nonstarchy vegetables such as broccoli and peppers.

(F) Removing the noodles removes most of the carbs, and the protein in beef is satiating.

(G) Mashed potatoes are a fast carb. Choose noodles and a mix of root vegetables, or roasted onions, mushrooms, or Brussels sprouts instead—the carbohydrate is held between an abundance of fiber, which slows it down.

(H) Removing the noodles removes most of the carbs. Be generous with the root vegetables to ensure you do not feel deprived.

Friday

	FAST CARBS	SLOW CARBS	LOW CARBS
Breakfast	Toasted white bread, butter, and fried egg Flavored latte	Chicken, spinach, and onion omelet on a small slice of whole grain bread (A) Coffee with cream (B)	Chicken, spinach, onion, and cheese omelet (C) Black coffee (D)
Lunch	Pita bread and chicken with side salad	Grilled chicken and quinoa salad (E)	Grilled chicken salad with grated cheese and pine nuts (F)
Dinner	Chicken and mushroom risotto (made with regular risotto rice)	Chicken and mushroom risotto (made with buckwheat) (G)	Chicken and mushroom risotto (made with cauliflower) (H)

(A) Instead of having fried eggs with white bread, choose a small slice of whole grain bread and add in nonstarchy vegetables such as spinach and onion.

(B) Flavored drinks from coffeehouses often contain a lot of added sugar, and all that milk—whether regular or alternative varieties like oat or almond—may contain a good deal of carbs as well. (Some almond milks are low in carbs.) Skip the coffee concoctions and opt for brewed coffee with a splash of cream.

(C) Removing the bread removes most of the carbs. Add cheese to the omelet for protein and fat.

(D) The lowest carb coffee option is to simply drink it black.

(E) The glycemic index of pita breads varies. Choose an intact grain such as quinoa to accompany the salad instead.

(F) Removing the quinoa removes most of the carbs. Add some grated cheese and pine nuts for protein, fat, and flavor.

(G) Slow down the carbs in risotto by substituting the rice with buckwheat. Buckwheat takes longer to digest than rice so the carbs are released more slowly.

(H) Removing the risotto removes most of the carbs. Try cauliflower risotto instead, which is made with cauliflower rice (available in the frozen foods section of most grocery stores).

Saturday

	FAST CARBS	SLOW CARBS	LOW CARBS
Breakfast	Breakfast smoothie: oats, banana, milk, strawberries, and almonds blended	Whole oats with chopped strawberries and whole almonds (A)	Low-carb muesli made with unsweetened coconut flakes, sliced almond, and mixed seeds; sliced strawberries (B)
Lunch	BBQ chicken wings and french fries Raspberry sorbet	Grilled fish and coleslaw (C) Frozen yogurt with sliced strawberries (D)	Grilled fish and coleslaw Greek yogurt with sliced strawberries (E)
Dinner	Beef with rice and vegetables	Beef with beans (F) and vegetables	Beef with vegetables with a generous drizzle of olive or canola oil (G)

(A) Smoothies have a reputation for being healthy. The blender, however, does the body's work for it: think of the blender as "predigesting" your food. Eat the carbs in the oats, fruit, and nuts whole to keep them slow.

(B) You can make your own low-carb muesli from unsweetened coconut flakes and a mixture of sliced nuts and seeds. There are many recipes online you can try for this and other menu items.

(C) Instead of fast carbs from potatoes, choose coleslaw made with a variety of slow- and high-fiber carbs including raisins, cabbage, fennel, and celery root.

(D) Instead of sorbet, which is a fast carb, choose frozen yogurt with strawberry slices. Some frozen yogurts are high in sugar, but the protein and fat in the yogurt helps slow down the carbs.

(E) For a low-carb dessert, have plain Greek yogurt, which has no added sugar, with sliced strawberries.

(F) Instead of rice, choose a legume such as cannellini beans or chickpeas. The carbs in legumes are harder for the body to break down, so they are released more slowly.

(G) By removing the beans, you remove most of the carbs. Add extra vegetables and a generous drizzle of a healthy oil to help you stay full.

Sunday

	FAST CARBS	SLOW CARBS	LOW CARBS
Breakfast	Cereal bar Fruit smoothie: kiwis, strawberries, banana	Homemade whole cereal with oat flakes, sunflower seeds, and hazelnuts (A) Whole banana (B)	Homemade whole cereal with shredded coconut, sunflower seeds, and hazelnuts (C) Kiwi fruit (D)
Lunch	Rice cakes with cottage cheese and smoked salmon	Smoked salmon with barley salad (E)	Smoked salmon with leafy green salad topped with avocado and pine nuts (F)
Dinner	Pork, sticky rice, and vegetables	Pork, udon noodles, and vegetables (G)	Pork, broccoli, and zucchini noodles (H)

(A) Cereal bars are often marketed as healthy but usually contain processed cereal grains with added sugars. Make your own cereal with plain steel-cut oats and whole nuts and seeds such as hazelnuts and sunflower seeds.

(B) Fruit smoothies are high in sugar—they contain far more fruit than you would normally eat whole. In addition, the skins and seeds are typically removed, which strips away plant fiber. Choose a small serving of whole fruit instead.

(C) As mentioned, by removing the oats, you remove most of the carbs. Make your own low-carb muesli from unsweetened coconut flakes and a mixture of sliced nuts and seeds.

(D) Depending on your desired carb limit, replacing a whole banana with a kiwi fruit can lower the carb content by more than ten grams.

(E) Rice cakes are a fast carb. Choose an intact grain such as a salad made with barley for a slow-carb alternative.

(F) By removing the barley, you remove most of the carbs. Add a large serving of leafy green salad with added avocado and pine nuts for healthy, satisfying fats.

(G) Sticky, or gelatinous, rice is the "fastest" kind of rice. In contrast, noodles such as udon noodles contain slower carbs.

(H) By removing the noodles, you remove most of the carbs. Try swapping in a vegetable-based noodle instead, like zucchini noodles or sweet potato noodles.

Q&A

Q&A with Dr. Nicola Guess—About the Menus

DK: Can you explain what you have done with these menus?

NG: As you have written, in most Western countries, people get far too many calories from processed "fast" carbs. Reducing the amount of fast carbs in the diet will improve health, but how to do this will depend on personal choice. I have given a few options. For example, a person could choose to simply switch from a fast carb to a slow carb. Some people may choose to avoid starchy carbs entirely. Most people who do this find that adding a little extra protein or healthy fats can ensure they feel full while managing their weight. I have shown both these approaches. Alternatively, one could choose to replace the fast carb with a combination of protein and slow carbs. The consistent theme here is reducing or avoiding fast carbs.

DK: Which fast carbs do you see as the biggest problems in American diets?

NG: Bread, breakfast cereal, and sugary drinks like soda. The first two represent a large proportion of the carbohydrate intake of Americans. Not only that, those two are particularly problematic because many people believe them to be healthy. These products are marketed in such a way that consumers see "whole grain" or "high fiber" on the package and think they're making a wholesome choice. As you have shown, they're not.

Soda is an obvious problem. As everyone knows, it's full of sugar. Adolescents, for example, can get up to a quarter of their calories from soda. For lots of people, the single most effective dietary change is simple: stop drinking liquid sugar.

DK: How has this information influenced how you designed the meals in these menus? Let's start with breakfast.

NG: You'll notice in the Monday example, the commercial breakfast cereal, Cheerios, has been switched to whole intact oats. Whether the oats are steel cut or rolled doesn't really make a difference—the important thing is that both of these varieties have the outside layer of the grain, the really fibrous part, intact. This is in contrast to the oats in Cheerios—milled, mashed, and processed beyond recognition. Some people find oats plain or boring on their own, but to add texture and sweetness, you can add in some whole fruit or nuts and seeds. You'll notice I've added whole blueberries in place of the blueberry puree from concentrate found in the Cheerios. But you could add any fruit you enjoy, such as berries or bananas.

DK: That's a really simple switch!

NG: It is, and one of the things I always reiterate to my patients is that you have to be savvy about food marketing. Lots of commercial cereals are marketed as whole grain, yet, as you've written, "whole grain" is a marketing term and does not necessarily mean intact. All intact grains are whole grains, but not all whole grains are intact.

What's even more confusing for consumers is when fiber is added after intensive processing. As you have pointed out, we know scientifically this does not mimic the effect of naturally intact grains on our bodies, but right now there's no way of determining this from nutrition labels. In fact, compare the fiber content of whole oats and Cheerios: about seven to eight grams of fiber per hundred grams of product in each. How would the consumer know the difference? So I always let my patients know to look for steel cut or rolled oats (they might also be labeled as Scottish oats in the supermarket), but not instant oats.

DK: What about any other fast carbs in breakfasts?

NG: I have included toast in day two. The fast carb, white bread, has been replaced by pumpernickel bread. Choosing a slow replacement isn't easy. Many commercial whole grain breads undergo the same problematic method of processing as cereals: the whole grain is broken down and then the milled fiber is added back in. It's not immediately obvious from the label that this is the case. So a better option is to choose rye or pumpernickel breads. Rye is unusual because it has fiber in the endosperm as well as the bran. An authentic pumpernickel bread should have rye flour as the first ingredient, and typically the flour is coarsely ground (less processed). Look for whole grain rye on the ingredients list. Watch out for imitations, which have wheat flour as the first ingredient, a small amount of the beneficial rye flour, and then add caramel coloring to fool you.

DK: I can also see that where fruit juice or smoothies appear in the fast carbs section, you have switched to the whole fruit. Can you explain why that is?

NG: Lots of people consider fruit juices to be a healthy choice. In fact, some people think of fruit in liquid form as healthier than whole fruit, but typically a fruit smoothie could contain six to seven servings of fruit. And that is the problem. Fruit does contain naturally occurring sugar, which is usually a mixture of fructose, sucrose, and glucose. Some fruits, such as bananas, also contain some starch. The amount of these sugars might be as little as three to four grams in a serving of strawberries, or perhaps up to fifteen grams in the case of an apple or mango. And remember, the sugar here is coming with a lot of fiber and other beneficial nutrients. So think about what happens when you add six or seven fruits into a blender or juicer—you can easily have forty to sixty grams of sugar in an eight- to ten-ounce serving.

We also know that, for reasons we don't fully understand, sugar in liquid form is worse for our metabolic health than the same amount of sugar in a solid food. Then there is the processing itself, and the fact that some fruit juices or smoothies actually remove the fibrous pulp. Then finally, many fruit drinks contain added sugar. Some of the strongest and most consistent advice we should be giving as health professionals is to eat the whole fruit. Treat smoothies and fruit juices as you would Coca-Cola—avoid or have as an occasional treat.

DK: Can you give us other examples of how you've switched from fast to slow carbs in the menus?

NG: One thing a lot of people don't know is that pasta may be a healthier choice than rice because a lot of the starch in pasta is "resistant starch." And the starch becomes even more resistant if you cook and cool the pasta. And of course, resistant starch is a slow carb. So a cold pasta salad is a great choice.

Another great addition to meals—and pretty easy to do—is to use more pulses, foods such as chickpeas, lentils, and beans. They're cheap, full of phytonutrients and fiber, and also a good source of protein. You can see in the menu, I have replaced rice (a fast carb) with beans to serve with vegetables alongside some beef.

In addition, by switching from white rice to basmati rice, you can slow the carbs down. An even better change is to reduce the serving size of basmati rice and add lentils. That way, you still get your rice in the meal, but you're also adding nutrition-rich lentils and slowing the carbs down even more. That kind of meal will keep you satisfied much longer than the one containing the usual white rice.

You'll also notice I have used a variety of whole grains. These are grains like buckwheat, quinoa, and bulgur wheat. These are intact grains which can be used in salads or as a replacement for a slow-carb risotto.

DK: Let's look at the low-carb menu items. You haven't just taken out the carb; you've replaced it with something else.

NG: As you have demonstrated, some people find that a low-carbohydrate diet can be an effective way to lose weight. While the initial weight loss itself is relatively easy to achieve, the real challenge lies in maintaining the weight loss. With many diets, the hunger kicks in, people eat more, and they regain the weight. What you're looking to achieve is a physiologically, psychologically, and socially satisfying diet. You have shown that adding in high-fiber foods and protein can help increase fullness hormones (e.g., GLP-1) and keep us fuller for longer. But let's not forget the social and psychological issues around meals. It can be hard, given the way we may be used to eating, to look at a plate of only a chicken breast with a few tomatoes and some lettuce. And you also don't want to have a meal that you eat so quickly that you've finished long before everyone else at the table. So you can see each low-carb meal includes lots of nonstarchy veggies. You can also see that I've added in nuts and seeds for the fiber, protein, and healthy fats, but also for texture and taste. I've also added in some cheese—this is high in protein. I've also included a generous serving of olive oil in many of the meals. Putting all this together, you get a meal which covers the whole plate—so you don't feel deprived. The meals also have a variety of taste and textures to keep you satisfied, but none of the starchy carbohydrate.

DK: I can see you still have included fruit in the low-carb meals, though.

NG: If someone is eating a full meal high in healthy fat, fiber, and protein, and then has a small amount of fruit for dessert, in most people this will have an insignificant effect on blood glucose or insulin. For many people with prediabetes or type 2 diabetes, they might choose to avoid certain fruits which they find drive up their glucose, and this is fine. Many of my patients with type 2 diabetes choose lower sugar fruits such as berries or avocado. But I think an important message we do need to get out there, especially for people who don't have diabetes, is that fruit is not a problem in moderation.

Notes

Introduction: The Birth of Fast Carbs

Sources
Works Referenced

Franck, Caroline, Sonia M. Grandi, and Mark J. Eisenberg. "Agricultural Subsidies and the American Obesity Epidemic." *American Journal of Preventive Medicine* 45, no. 3 (September 2013): 327–33, doi:10.1016/j.amepre.2013.04.010.

"From George Washington to Lafayette, 18 June 1788," *Founders Online,* National Archives, https://founders.archives.gov/documents/Washington/04-06-02-0301 (accessed October 30, 2019).

George Washington's Mount Vernon. "Mansion." https://www.mountvernon.org/the-estate-gardens/the-mansion/.

Global Food Forum. 2018 Clean Label Conference. Itasca, IL, March 27, 2018.

"The Hatch Act of 1887." North Dakota State University Library, NDSU Repository, https://library.ndsu.edu/ir/bitstream/handle/10365/6113/farm_45_03_01.pdf?sequence=1&isAllowed=y.

MacLean, Eliza. "American Agricultural Policy: How Food Shaped the United States." *U.S. History Scene,* April 10, 2015, http://ushistoryscene.com/article/ag-policy/.

Interviews and Correspondence with the Author

Fitzgerald, Kate (June 2019). I am indebted to Kate Fitzgerald, who provided invaluable insight into the history of agricultural policy in the United States.

Notes

xv **"storehouse and granary":** "From George Washington to Lafayette."

xvii **"clean" and "natural":** Dave Lundahl and Sarah Kirkmeyer, "Tapping into the Implicit Minds of Clean Label Enthusiasts: Faster, More Consumer-Driven Ingredient Decisions"; Cara Newkirk, "Understanding the 'Clean Balancer' Consumer"; Donna Klockeman, "Hydrocolloid and Sweetener Alternatives: A Holistic Approach to Reformulation"; and Steve Peirce, "Clean Label Ingredient Alternatives." All lectures presented at the Institute of Food Technologists, IFT 18 Clean Label Product Development: Balancing Consumer, Regulatory, and Science, Chicago, IL, July 15, 2018.

Chapter 1: An extraordinary opportunity to save lives

Sources
Works Referenced

GBD 2017 Diet Collaborators. "Health Effects of Dietary Risks in 195 Countries, 1990–2017: A Systematic Analysis for the Global Burden of Disease Study 2017." *Lancet* 393, no. 10184 (May 11, 2019): 1958–72.

Interviews and Correspondence with the Author

Fitzgerald, Kate (June 2019).

Notes

4   **eleven million deaths:** GBD 2017 Diet Collaborators, "Health Effects of Dietary Risks in 195 Countries."

Chapter 2: There is a path out of the lifelong trap of food chaos that leads to lasting weight loss and health

Sources
Works Referenced

Kessler, David A. *The End of Overeating: Taking Control of the Insatiable American Appetite.* New York: Rodale, 2009.

———. "The Evolution of National Nutrition Policy." *Annual Review of Nutrition* 15 (July 1995): xiii–xxvi.

————. *A Question of Intent: A Great American Battle with a Deadly Industry*. New York: PublicAffairs, 2001.

Kessler, David A., Jerold R. Mande, F. Edward Scarbrough, Renie Schapiro, and Karyn Feiden. "Developing the 'Nutrition Facts' Food Label." *Harvard Health Policy Review* 4, no. 2 (Fall 2003): 13–24.

National Center for Health Statistics. *Health, United States, 2017*. Hyattsville, MD: U.S. Department of Health and Human Services, 2018.

Notes

9   **More than two-thirds of Americans:** National Center for Health Statistics, 10.

10   **The book I wrote:** Kessler, *End of Overeating*.

12   **I had helped design:** Kessler, "Evolution of National Nutrition Policy"; Kessler, *Question of Intent*; Kessler et al., "Developing the 'Nutrition Facts' Food Label."

Chapter 3: Until we learn the truth about fast carbs, we won't break the weight loss-and-gain cycle

Sources
Works Referenced

Furness, John B., Leni R. Rivera, Hyun-Jung Cho, David M. Bravo, and Brid Callaghan. "The Gut as a Sensory Organ." *Nature Reviews Gastroenterology & Hepatology* 10, no. 12 (September 24, 2013): 729–40, doi:10.1038/nrgastro.2013.180.

Chapter 4: The problem posed by highly processed (fast) carbs has been suspected for decades

Sources
Works Referenced

Chestnut, Glenn F. *Father Ed Dowling: Bill Wilson's Sponsor*. Bloomington, IN: iUniverse Books, 2015.

Dowling, Edward J. "A.A. Steps for the Underprivileged Non-A.A." In Robert Fitzgerald, *The Soul of Sponsorship: The Friendship of Fr. Ed*

Dowling, S.J. and Bill Wilson in Letters, 125–28. Center City, MN: Hazelden, 1995.

Graham, Sylvester. *A Treatise on Bread and Bread-Making.* American Antiquarian Cookbook Collection. Ed. American Antiquarian Society. 1837; Kansas City, MO: Andrews McMeel Publishing, 2012.

S., Rozanne. *Beyond Our Wildest Dreams: A History of Overeaters Anonymous as Seen by a Cofounder.* Rio Rancho, NM: Overeaters Anonymous, 1996.

Notes

16   **In 1837, the preacher:** Graham, *Treatise on Bread.*

17   **"My 240-pound gluttony":** Dowling, "A.A. Steps," 126.

Chapter 5: Only 12.2 percent of Americans are metabolically healthy

Sources
Works Referenced

Araujo, Joana, Jianwen Cai, and June Stevens. "Only 12.5% of American Adults Are Metabolically Healthy—NHANES 2009–2016." Lecture presented at ObesityWeek presented by The Obesity Society (TOS) in partnership with the American Society for Metabolic and Bariatric Surgery (ASMBS), Nashville, TN, November 13, 2018.

———. "Prevalence of Optimal Metabolic Health in American Adults: National Health and Nutrition Examination Survey 2009–2016." *Metabolic Syndrome and Related Disorders* 17, no. 1 (February 2019): 46–52, https://doi.org/10.1089/met.2018.0105.

Bays, Harold. "Adiposopathy, 'Sick Fat,' Ockham's Razor, and Resolution of the Obesity Paradox." *Current Atherosclerosis Reports* 16, no. 5 (2014): 409, https://doi.org/10.1007/s11883-014-0409-1.

———. "The Future of Obesity Medicine: Managing Adiposity-Related Disease with Obesity Treatment." Lecture delivered at the Spring Obesity Summit 2019, Phoenix, AZ, April 5, 2019.

Notes

19   **only 12.2 percent of Americans:** Araujo, Cai, and Stevens, "Prevalence of Optimal Metabolic Health in American Adults."

20   **"When you increase body fat":** Bays, "Future of Obesity Medicine."

Chapter 6: Over the past half century, Americans have greatly increased their average daily intake of processed carbohydrates

Sources
Works Referenced

Fryar, C. D., Q. Gu, C. L. Ogden, and K. M. Flegal. "Anthropometric Reference Data for Children and Adults: United States, 2011–2014." National Center for Health Statistics. *Vital Health Statistics* 3, no. 39 (2016), https://stacks.cdc.gov/view/cdc/40572.

Kessler, David A. *The End of Overeating: Taking Control of the Insatiable American Appetite.* New York: Rodale, 2009.

Ogden, Cynthia L., and Margaret D. Carroll. "Prevalence of Overweight, Obesity, and Extreme Obesity among Adults: United States, Trends 1960–1962 through 2007–2008." Centers for Disease Control and Prevention, https://www.cdc.gov/nchs/data/hestat/obesity_adult_07_08/obesity_adult_07_08.htm (accessed August 28, 2019).

Ogden, C. L., C. D. Fryar, M. D. Carroll, and K. M. Flegal. "Mean Body Weight, Height, and Body Mass, United States, 1960–2002." *Advance Data from Vital and Health Statistics* no. 347. Hyattsville, MD: National Center for Health Statistics, 2004.

Steele, Eurídice Martínez, Larissa Galastri Baraldi, Maria Laura da Costa Louzada, Jean-Claude Moubarac, et al. "Ultra-Processed Foods and Added Sugars in the US Diet: Evidence from a Nationally Representative Cross-Sectional Study." *BMJ Open* 6 (2016): e009892, doi: 10.1136/bmjopen-2015-009892.

United States Department of Agriculture. "Food Availability (Per Capita) Data System, Data Set: Calories.xls." Washington, DC: Economic Research Service, 2019, https://www.ers.usda.gov/data-products/food-availability-per-capita-data-system/.

Interviews and Correspondence with the Author

Buzby, Jean C. (Jan. 2019)

Jones, Julie Miller (July 2018)

Tosh, Susan (Oct. 2018)

Notes

25 **shift began in the 1970s:** Fryar et al., "Anthropometric Reference Data."

26 **about twenty pounds heavier:** Kessler, *End of Overeating*; Ogden and Carroll, "Prevalence of Overweight."

Chapter 7: A turning point for our diet

Sources
Works Referenced

"The Fat of the Land." *Time*, January 13, 1961, 48.

Hunger in America. Produced by Martin Carr. CBS News, May 21, 1968. TV documentary.

Lasby, Clarence G. *Eisenhower's Heart Attack: How Ike Beat Heart Disease and Held on to the Presidency*. Lawrence: University Press of Kansas, 1997.

Oppenheimer, Gerald M., and I. Daniel Benrubi. "McGovern's Senate Select Committee on Nutrition and Human Needs versus the Meat Industry on the Diet-Heart Question (1976–1977)." *American Journal of Public Health* 104, no. 1 (January 2014): 59–69, https://www.ncbi.nlm.nih.gov/pubmed/24228658.

United States. Congress. Senate. Select Committee on Nutrition and Human Needs. *Compilation of the National School Lunch Act and the Child Nutrition Act of 1966: With Related Provisions of Law and Authorities for Commodities Distribution*. Washington, DC: GPO, December 1974, https://catalog.hathitrust.org/Record/003217990.

———. *Diet Related to Killer Diseases: Hearings before the Select Committee on Nutrition and Human Needs of the United States Senate, Ninety-Fourth Congress, Second Session, July 27 and 28, 1976*. Washington, DC: GPO, 1976, http://catalog.hathitrust.org/Record/007401470.

————. *Diet Related to Killer Diseases II: Hearings before the Select Committee on Nutrition and Human Needs of the United States Senate, Ninety-Fifth Congress, First Session, February 1 and 2, 1977.* Washington, DC: GPO, 1977, http://catalog.hathitrust.org/Record/007418251.

————. *Diet Related to Killer Diseases III: Hearings before the Select Committee on Nutrition and Human Needs of the United States Senate, Ninety-Fifth Congress, First Session, March 24, 1977.* Washington, DC: GPO, 1977, https://catalog.hathitrust.org/Record/012480120.

————. *Diet Related to Killer Diseases IV: Hearings before the Select Committee on Nutrition and Human Needs of the United States Senate, Ninety-Fifth Congress, First Session, March 31, 1977. Dietary Fiber and Health.* Washington, DC: GPO, 1977, https://catalog.hathitrust.org/Record/01248 0155.

————. *Diet Related to Killer Diseases VIII: Hearings before the Select Committee on Nutrition and Human Needs of the United States Senate, Ninety-Fifth Congress, First Session, October 17, 1977. HEW Overview.* Washington, DC: GPO, 1977, https://catalog.hathitrust.org/Record/01248 0158.

————. *Dietary Goals for the United States.* 2nd ed. Washington, DC: GPO, December 1977, http://hdl.handle.net/2027/uiug.30112023368936.

Interviews and Correspondence with the Author

Matz, Marshall L. (Nov. 2018, Jan. 2019)

Notes

28   **CBS documentary:** *Hunger in America.*

29   **goal of the McGovern Committee:** Oppenheimer and Benrubi, "McGovern's Senate Select Committee."

29   **McGovern stated confidently:** U.S. Senate Select Committee on Nutrition and Human Needs, *Dietary Goals for the United States.*

29   **stress the links:** Ibid.

30   **testified that obesity:** Ibid., xvii–xviii.

30   **1961 cover of *Time*:** "Fat of the Land."

Chapter 8: Government guidelines led us to carbs

Sources
Works Referenced

United States. Congress. Senate. Select Committee on Nutrition and Human Needs. *Dietary Goals for the United States.* 2nd ed. Washington, DC: GPO, 1977 (December), http://hdl.handle.net/2027/uiug.30112023368936.

———. *Dietary Goals for the United States Prepared by the Staff of the Select Committee on Nutrition and Human Needs, United States Senate.* Washington, DC: GPO, 1977 (February), http://hdl.handle.net/2027/umn.31951d00283419d.

———. *Diet and Killer Diseases with Press Reaction and Additional Information.* Washington, DC: GPO, 1977.

Notes

32 ***Dietary Goals for the United States*:** U.S. Senate Select Committee on Nutrition and Human Needs, *Dietary Goals for the United States Prepared by the Staff of the Select Committee.*

32 **Hegsted encouraged Americans:** U.S. Senate Select Committee on Nutrition and Human Needs, *Diet and Killer Diseases,* 209.

32 **expressed doubt about:** U.S. Senate Select Committee on Nutrition and Human Needs, *Dietary Goals for the United States,* 2nd ed., xxiii.

33 **[Hegsted] . . . pushed for decisive recommendations:** U.S. Senate Select Committee on Nutrition and Human Needs, *Diet and Killer Diseases,* 209.

33 **actually proposed in the guidelines:** U.S. Senate Select Committee on Nutrition and Human Needs, *Dietary Goals for the United States Prepared by the Staff of the Select Committee,* 14–51.

34 **"Bread is of intermediate caloric density":** U.S. Senate Select Committee on Nutrition and Human Needs, *Dietary Goals for the United States,* 2nd ed., 21.

34   **main disadvantage of white flour:** U.S. Senate Select Committee on Nutrition and Human Needs, *Dietary Goals for the United States Prepared by the Staff of the Select Committee*, 221, 229.

34   **white flour was "enriched":** Ibid., 42.

Chapter 9: "Complex carbohydrates" is a misleading term that fails to distinguish rapidly absorbable carbs from those we absorb slowly

Sources
Works Referenced

Cho, Susan Sungsoo. *Handbook of Dietary Fiber*. Food Science and Technology, vol. 113. New York: Marcel Dekker, 2001.

"Dietary Guidelines." U.S. Office of Disease Prevention and Health Promotion, https://health.gov/dietaryguidelines (accessed November 6, 2019).

Dobbing, John. *Dietary Starches and Sugars in Man: A Comparison*. ILSI Human Nutrition Reviews. London: Springer London, 1989.

Dona, Anthony C., Guilhem Pages, Robert G. Gilbert, and Philip W. Kuchel. "Digestion of Starch: In Vivo and In Vitro Kinetic Models Used to Characterise Oligosaccharide or Glucose Release." *Carbohydrate Polymers* 80, no. 3 (May 5, 2010): 599–617, doi:10.1016/j.carbpol.2010.01.002.

Dreher, Mark L., Claudia J. Dreher, James W. Berry, and Sharon E. Fleming. "Starch Digestibility of Foods: A Nutritional Perspective." *Critical Reviews in Food Science and Nutrition* 20, no. 1 (January 1984): 47–71, doi:10.1080/10408398409527383.

FAO. *Carbohydrates in Human Nutrition*. Food and Nutrition Paper, no. 66 (Rome: FAO, 1998).

Gunaratne, A., and H. Corke. "Starch, Analysis of Quality." *Reference Module in Food Science* (2016), doi:10.1016/b978-0-08-100596-5.00092-5.

Madhusudhan, Basavaraj, and Rudrapatnam N. Tharanathan. "Legume and Cereal Starches: Why Differences in Digestibility? Part 1: Isolation and Composition of Legume (Greengram and Bengalgram) Starches." *Starch–Stärke* 47, no. 5 (1995): 165–71, doi:10.1002/star.19950470502.

Singh, Jaspreet, Lovedeep Kaur, and Harjinder Singh. "Food Micro-structure and Starch Digestion." *Advances in Food and Nutrition Research* (2013): 137–79, doi:10.1016/b978-0-12-416555-7.00004-7.

Svihus, B., A. K. Uhlen, and O. M. Harstad. "Effect of Starch Granule Structure, Associated Components and Processing on Nutritive Value of Cereal Starch: A Review." *Animal Feed Science and Technology* 122, no. 3–4 (September 2005): 303–20, doi:10.1016/j.anifeedsci.2005.02.025.

Tester, Richard F., John Karkalas, and Xin Qi. "Starch—Composition, Fine Structure and Architecture." *Journal of Cereal Science* 39, no. 2 (March 2004): 151–65, doi:10.1016/j.jcs.2003.12.001.

Chapter 10: Today's ultraprocessed foods allow us to absorb more calories

Sources
Works Referenced

Boback, Scott M., Christian L. Cox, Brian D. Ott, Rachel Carmody, et al. "Cooking and Grinding Reduces the Cost of Meat Digestion." *Comparative Biochemistry and Physiology, Part A* 148, no. 3 (2007): 651–56, https://www.sciencedirect.com/science/article/pii/S1095643307015632.

Carmody, Rachel N., Georg K. Gerber, Jesus M. Luevano, Daniel M. Gatti, et al. "Diet Dominates Host Genotype in Shaping the Murine Gut Microbiota." *Cell Host & Microbe* 17, no. 1 (2015): 72–84, https://www.sciencedirect.com/science/article/pii/S1931312814004260.

Carmody, Rachel N., Gil S. Weintraub, and Richard W. Wrangham. "Energetic Consequences of Thermal and Nonthermal Food Processing." *Proceedings of the National Academy of Sciences of the United States of America* 108, no. 48 (2011): 19199–203, https://www.jstor.org/stable/23066741.

Carmody, Rachel N., and Richard W. Wrangham. "The Energetic Significance of Cooking." *Journal of Human Evolution* 57, no.4 (2009): 379–91, https://www.sciencedirect.com/science/article/pii/S0047248409001262.

———. "Our Nutrition Labels Are Lying about How Many Calories Foods Have." *Washington Post*, January 6, 2015.

David, Lawrence A., Corinne F. Maurice, Rachel N. Carmody, David B. Gootenberg, et al. "Diet Rapidly and Reproducibly Alters the Human Gut

Microbiome." *Nature* 505, no. 7484 (2014): 559–63, https://www.ncbi
.nlm.nih.gov/pubmed/24336217.

Wrangham, Richard, and Rachel Carmody. "Human Adaptation to the
Control of Fire." *Evolutionary Anthropology: Issues, News, and Reviews* 19,
no. 5 (2010): 187–99, doi:10.1002/evan.20275.

Interviews and Correspondence with the Author

Anonymous food designer

Notes

40   **"labels ignore the costs":** Carmody and Wrangham, "Our Nutrition Labels Are Lying."

Chapter 11: The food industry claims there are no negative effects to processing

Sources
Works Referenced

Clemens, Roger. "Impact of Processing on Nutrition." Lecture delivered
in four sections as part of the Institute of Food Technologists' "Food
Science for the Non-Food Scientist" online course, https://www.pathlms
.com/ift-learn-online/courses/1806/sections/2304 (accessed November 8,
2019).

———. "The Role of Processed Foods in Delivering Nutrition." Lecture
delivered at the Institute of Food Technologists, IFT 18 Clean Label Product Development: Balancing Consumer, Regulatory, and Science, Chicago, IL, July 16–18, 2018.

Institute of Food Technologists. "IFT—Feeding the Future," www.ift.org
/about-ift (accessed November 10, 2019).

International Nut and Dried Fruit Council. "Traditional Dried Fruits:
Valuable Tools to Meet Dietary Recommendations for Fruit Intake," 2011,
https://www.nutfruit.org/consumers/news/detail/traditional-dried-fruits
-valuable-tools-to-meet-dietary-recommendations-for-fruit-intake.

Monteiro, Carlos Augusto, Geoffrey Cannon, Jean-Claude Moubarac, Renata Bertazzi Levy, et al. "The UN Decade of Nutrition, the NOVA Food

Classification, and the Trouble with Ultra-Processing." *Public Health Nutrition* 21, no. 1 (March 21, 2017): 5–17, doi:10.1017/s1368980017000234.

Sadler, Michele Jeanne, Sigrid Gibson, Kevin Whelan, Marie-Ann Ha, et al. "Dried Fruit and Public Health: What Does the Evidence Tell Us?" *International Journal of Food Sciences and Nutrition* 70, no. 6 (February 27, 2019): 675–87, doi:10.1080/09637486.2019.1568398.

Interviews and Correspondence with the Author

BeMiller, James N. (Jan. 2019)

Notes

41 **"safe, nutritious, and sustainable":** Institute of Food Technologists.

42 **"deliberate practices":** Clemens, "Impact of Processing on Nutrition" and "Role of Processed Foods" (from slides presented at lectures and available to attendees and online participants or for purchase via IFT).

43 **"antioxidants are concentrated":** International Nut and Dried Fruit Council, cited in Clemens, "Impact of Processing on Nutrition" and "Role of Processed Foods."

44 **"hyper-palatable and attractive":** Monteiro et al, "UN Decade of Nutrition."

Chapter 12: From whole grain to the cereal box: What are we really eating?

Sources
Works Referenced

Crosbie, Graham B., and Andrew S. Ross. *The RVA Handbook*. St. Paul, MN: American Association of Cereal Chemists, 2007.

Delcour, Jan A., and R. Carl Hoseney. *Principles of Cereal Science and Technology*. 3rd ed. St. Paul, MN: American Association of Cereal Chemists, 2010.

Eliasson, Ann-Charlotte, ed. *Starch in Food*. Boca Raton, FL: CRC Press, 2004.

Fast, Robert B., and Elwood F. Caldwell, eds. *Breakfast Cereals and How They Are Made*. St. Paul, MN: American Association of Cereal Chemists, 2000.

Guine, Raquel de Pinho Ferreira, and Paula Maria dos Reis Correia, eds. *Engineering Aspects of Cereal and Cereal-Based Products*. Boca Raton, FL: CRC Press, 2014.

Kaletunc, Gonul, and Kenneth J. Breslauer, eds. *Characterization of Cereals and Flours: Properties, Analysis, and Applications*. Boca Raton, FL: CRC Press, 2003.

Kulp, Karel, and Joseph G. Ponte Jr., eds. *Handbook of Cereal Science and Technology*. 2nd ed., rev. and exp. New York: Marcel Dekker, 2000.

Marquart, Len, David R. Jacobs, Graeme H. McIntosh, Kaisa Poutanen, and Marla Reicks, eds. *Whole Grains and Health*. Ames, IA: Blackwell, 2007.

Matz, Samuel A. *The Chemistry and Technology of Cereals as Food and Feed*. 2nd ed. New Delhi: Scientific International, 2014.

Moyer, Melinda Wenner. "Whole-Grain Foods Not Always Healthful." *Scientific American*, July 25, 2013, https://www.scientificamerican.com/article/whole-grain-foods-not-always-healthful.

Chapter 13: Food processing changes the chemical structure of starch

Sources
Works Referenced

Chinnaswamy, R., and M. A. Hanna. "Macromolecular and Functional Properties of Native and Extrusion-Cooked Corn Starch." *Cereal Chemistry* 67, no. 5 (1990): 490–99, https://www.aaccnet.org/publications/cc/backissues/1990/Documents/67_490.pdf.

Dreher, Mark L., Claudia J. Dreher, James W. Berry, and Sharon E. Fleming. "Starch Digestibility of Foods: A Nutritional Perspective." *CRC Critical Reviews in Food Science and Nutrition* 20, no. 1 (January 1984): 47–71, doi:10.1080/10408398409527383.

Einde, René van den. "Molecular Modification of Starch during Thermomechanical Treatment." Doctoral thesis, Wageningen University, 2004.

Forte, Dennis, and Gordon Young. *Food and Extrusion Technology: An Applied Approach to Extrusion Theory*. Brisbane, Australia: Food Industry Engineering, 2016.

Grayson, Amanda. "Invention Blasts Off Our Cereal Business." General Mills blog. October 17, 2013, https://blog.generalmills.com.

Guha, Manisha, and S. Zakiuddin Ali. "Molecular Degradation of Starch during Extrusion Cooking of Rice." *International Journal of Food Properties* 5, no. 3 (January 11, 2002): 509–21, doi:10.1081/jfp-12001 5488.

Guy, Robin. *Extrusion Cooking: Technologies and Applications.* Cambridge, UK: Woodhead, 2001.

Holm, Jörgen, Barbro Hagander, Inger Björck, Ann-Charlotte Eliasson, and Ingmar Lundquist. "The Effect of Various Thermal Processes on the Glycemic Response to Whole Grain Wheat Products in Humans and Rats." *Journal of Nutrition* 119, no. 11 (November 1, 1989): 1631–38, doi:10.1093/jn/119.11.1631.

Maskan, Medeni. *Advances in Food Extrusion Technology.* Boca Raton, FL: CRC Press, 2012.

Miller, Kevin. "Does Processing Grains Impact Nutrition?" Lecture presented at the 2018 Oldways Whole Grains Council Conference, Seattle, WA, November 5, 2018.

Moscicki, Leszek. *Extrusion-Cooking Techniques.* Lublin, Poland: Wiley–VCH Verlag & Co. KGaA, 2011.

Singh, Jaspreet, Anne Dartois, and Lovedeep Kaur. "Starch Digestibility in Food Matrix: A Review." *Trends in Food Science & Technology* 21, no. 4 (April 2010): 168–80, doi:10.1016/j.tifs.2009.12.001.

Svihus, B., A. K. Uhlen, and O. M. Harstad. "Effect of Starch Granule Structure, Associated Components and Processing on Nutritive Value of Cereal Starch: A Review." *Animal Feed Science and Technology* 122, no. 3–4 (September 2005): 303–20, doi:10.1016/j.anifeedsci.2005.02.025.

Tamura, Masatsugu, Jaspreet Singh, Lovedeep Kaur, and Yukiharu Ogawa. "Impact of the Degree of Cooking on Starch Digestibility of Rice: An In Vitro Study." *Food Chemistry* 191 (January 2016): 98–104, doi:10.1016/j.foodchem.2015.03.127.

White, G. A., F. J. Doucet, S. E. Hill, and J. Wiseman. "Physicochemical Changes to Starch Granules during Micronisation and Extrusion Processing of Wheat, and Their Implications for Starch Digestibility in the Newly Weaned Piglet." *Animal* 2, no. 9 (September 2008): 1312–23, doi:10.1017 /s1751731108002553.

Ye, Jiangping, Xiuting Hu, Shunjing Luo, Wei Liu, et al. "Properties of Starch after Extrusion: A Review." *Starch–Stärke* 70, no. 11–12 (March 25, 2018), doi:10.1002/star.201700110.

Zhang, Genyi, and Bruce R. Hamaker. "The Nutritional Property of Endosperm Starch and Its Contribution to the Health Benefits of Whole Grain Foods." *Critical Reviews in Food Science and Nutrition* 57, no. 18 (February 6, 2016): 3807–17, doi:10.1080/10408398.2015.113 0685.

Zhu, Li-Jia, Radhiah Shukri, Normell Jhoe de Mesa-Stonestreet, Sajid Alavi, et al. "Mechanical and Microstructural Properties of Soy Protein: High Amylose Corn Starch Extrudates in Relation to Physiochemical Changes of Starch during Extrusion." *Journal of Food Engineering* 100, no. 2 (2010): 232–38, https://www.sciencedirect.com/science/article/pii /S0260877410001858.

Interviews and Correspondence with the Author

BeMiller, James N. (Jan. 2019)

Hamaker, Bruce (Oct. 2018, June 2019)

Jane, Jay-Lin (Oct. 2018)

Scanlon, Martin (Oct. 2018)

Tosh, Susan (Oct. 2018)

Van Lengerich, Bernard (Nov. 2018)

Whalen, Paul (Nov. 2018)

Zhu, Li-Jia (Oct. 2018)

Notes

51 **"gun goes *boom*":** Grayson, "Invention Blasts Off Our Cereal Business" (referencing an unspecified 1940s *Fortune* magazine article).

Chapter 14: The altered structure of processed starch makes it a rapidly absorbable fast carb

Sources
Works Referenced

Cho, Susan Sungsoo. *Handbook of Dietary Fiber.* Food Science and Technology, vol. 113. New York: Marcel Dekker, 2001.

Englyst, Klaus N., and Hans N. Englyst. "Carbohydrate Bioavailability." *British Journal of Nutrition* 94, no. 1 (July 2005): 1–11, doi:10.1079/bjn 20051457.

Grundy, Myriam Marie-Louise. "Plant Cell Walls as Barriers to Lipid Bioaccesibility in Model Lipid-Rich Plant Food (Almond)." PhD thesis, King's College London, 2014.

Singh, Jaspreet, Thilo Berg, Allan Hardacre, and Mike J. Boland. "Cotyledon Cell Structure and *In Vitro* Starch Digestion in Navy Beans." In *Food Structures, Digestion and Health*, ed. Mike Boland, Matt Golding, and Harjinder Singh, 223–42. San Diego, CA: Elsevier Science, 2014.

Slavin, Joanne L. "Carbohydrates, Dietary Fiber, and Resistant Starch in White Vegetables: Links to Health Outcomes." *Advances in Nutrition* 4, no. 3 (2013): 351S–355S, https://www.ncbi.nlm.nih.gov/pubmed/2367 4804.

"Vegetables and Vegetable Products." *Food Chemistry* (n.d.): 770–79, doi: 10.1007/978-3-540-69934-7_18.

Wahlqvist, M. L., E. G. Wilmshurst, C. R. Murton, and E. N. Richardson. "The Effect of Chain Length on Glucose Absorption and the Related Metabolic Response." *American Journal of Clinical Nutrition* 31, no. 11 (November 1, 1978): 1998–2001, doi:10.1093/ajcn/31.11.1998.

Interviews and Correspondence with the Author

Björck, Inger (May 2019)

Hamaker, Bruce (Oct. 2018)

Chapter 15: Processed fast carbs serve as delivery vehicles for the pleasures of sugar, fat, and salt

Sources
Works Referenced

Erlanson-Albertsson, Charlotte. "How Palatable Food Disrupts Appetite Regulation." *Basic & Clinical Pharmacology & Toxicology* 97, no. 2 (August 2005): 61–73, doi:10.1111/j.1742-7843.2005.pto_179.x.

Here and Now Staff. "How the Food Industry Helps Engineer Our Cravings." NPR. December 16, 2015, https://www.npr.org/sections/the salt/2015/12/16/459981099/how-the-food-industry-helps-engineer-our -cravings.

Kessler, David A. *The End of Overeating: Taking Control of the Insatiable American Appetite.* New York: Rodale, 2009.

Miquel-Kergoat, S., V. Azais-Braesco, B. Burton-Freeman, and M. M. Hetherington. "Effects of Chewing on Appetite, Food Intake, and Gut Hormones: A Systematic Review and Meta-Analysis." *Physiology & Behavior* 151 (November 2015): 88–96, doi:10.1016/j.physbeh.2015.07 .017.

Interviews and Correspondence with the Author

Civille, Gail Vance (Nov. 2018, June 2019)

Chapter 16: Without processed starch, we would not have a vast array of processed foods

Sources
Works Referenced

Embuscado, Milda E. *Functionalizing Carbohydrates for Food Applications: Texturizing and Bioactive / Flavor Delivery Systems.* Lancaster, PA: Destech, 2014.

Korma, Sameh A., Kamal-Alahmad, Sobia Niazi, Al-Farga Ammar, et al. "Chemically Modified Starch and Utilization in Food Stuffs." *International Journal of Nutrition and Food Sciences* 5, no. 4 (2016): 264–72, doi:10.11648/j.ijnfs.20160504.15.

Lusas, Edmund W., and Lloyd W. Rooney. *Snack Foods Processing*. Lancaster, PA: Technomic, 2001.

Mouritsen, Ole G., and Klavs Styrbæk. *Mouthfeel: How Texture Makes Taste*. Trans. Mariela Johansen. New York: Columbia University Press, 2017.

Nieto Velez, Diana. "Formulating for Function: Winning Nutrition and Consumer Preference on Food Product Development Using Dietary Fiber, Hydrocolloid, and Starch." Lecture presented at Institute of Food Technologists, IFT 18 Clean Label Product Development: Balancing Consumer, Regulatory, and Science, Chicago, IL, July 16–18, 2018.

Payne, Charles Anthony. "The Use of Starch in Meat Products." PhD dissertation, Kansas State University, 1993.

Notes

61   **"starches in almost everything":** Nieto Velez, "Formulating for Function."

Chapter 17: Recommendation: reduce or eliminate fast carbs for good to achieve and maintain a healthy weight

Sources
Works Referenced

2018 Oldways Whole Grains Council Conference, Seattle, WA, November 4–6, 2018.

Ardent Mills. "Ultragrain Whole Wheat Flours," https://www.ardent mills.com/media/1083/ultragrain-whole-wheat-flours.pdf (accessed October 24, 2019).

Augustin, L. S. A., C. W. C. Kendall, D. J. A. Jenkins, W. C. Willett, et al. "Glycemic Index, Glycemic Load, and Glycemic Response: An International Scientific Consensus Summit from the International Carbohydrate Quality Consortium (ICQC)." *Nutrition, Metabolism and Cardiovascular Diseases* 25, no. 9 (2015): 795–815.

Aziz, Alfred. "The Glycemic Index: Methodological Aspects Related to the Interpretation of Health Effects and to Regulatory Labeling." *Journal of AOAC International* 92, no. 3 (May 2009): 879–87.

Aziz, Alfred, Lydia Dumais, and Jennifer Barber. "Health Canada's Evaluation of the Use of Glycemic Index Claims on Food Labels." *American Journal of Clinical Nutrition* 98, no. 2 (August 2013): 269–74.

Brand-Miller, Jennie, Joanna McMillan-Price, Katherine Steinbeck, and Ian Caterson. "Dietary Glycemic Index: Health Implications." *Journal of the American College of Nutrition* 28, suppl. 4 (August 2009): 446S–449S, doi:10.1080/07315724.2009.10718110.

Dodd, Hayley, Sheila Williams, Rachel Brown, and Bernard Venn. "Calculating Meal Glycemic Index by Using Measured and Published Food Values Compared with Directly Measured Meal Glycemic Index." *American Journal of Clinical Nutrition* 94, no. 4 (October 2011): 992–96.

Eades, Michael R. "Incretins, Insulin, and Food Quality." Lecture presented at Low Carb Conference, Denver, CO, March 7–10, 2019.

Englyst, Klaus N., and Hans N. Englyst. "Carbohydrate Bioavailability." *British Journal of Nutrition* 94, no. 1 (July 1, 2005): 1–11, doi:10.1079/bjn20051457.

Englyst, Klaus, Hans Englyst, Aurelie Goux, Alexandra Meynier, et al. "Inter-Laboratory Validation of the Starch Digestibility Method for Determination of Rapidly Digestible and Slowly Digestible Starch." *Food Chemistry* 245 (April 15, 2018): 1183–89.

Englyst, K. N., H. N. Englyst, G. J. Hudson, T. J. Cole, and J. H. Cummings. "Rapidly Available Glucose in Foods: An In Vitro Measurement That Reflects the Glycemic Response." *American Journal of Clinical Nutrition* 69, no. 3 (March 1999): 448–54.

Fatsecret. "100g Bagel: Nutrition Facts." August 21, 2007, www.fatsecret.com/calories-nutrition/generic/bagel?portionid=52220&portionamount=100.000.

Flint, Anne, Bente K. Møller, Anne Raben, Dorthe Pedersen, et al. "The Use of Glycaemic Index Tables to Predict Glycaemic Index of Composite Breakfast Meals." *British Journal of Nutrition* 91, no. 6 (June 1, 2004): 979–89.

Golay, A., A. M. Coulston, C. B. Hollenbeck, L. L. Kaiser, et al. "Comparison of Metabolic Effects of White Beans Processed into Two Different Physical Forms." *Diabetes Care* 9, no. 3 (May 1, 1986): 260–66.

Grant, Shannan M., and Thomas M. S. Wolever. "Perceived Barriers to Application of Glycaemic Index: Valid Concerns or Lost in Translation?" *Nutrients* 3, no. 3 (March 2011): 330–40.

Haber, G. B., K. W. Heaton, D. Murphy, and L. F. Burroughs. "Depletion and Disruption of Dietary Fibre: Effects on Satiety, Plasma-Glucose, and Serum-Insulin." *Lancet* 310, no. 8040 (1977): 679–82.

Hamaker, Bruce, Mario Martinez, Marwa El-Hindaway, and Fang Fang. "Carbohydrate Structure, Digestion, and Physiological Effects." Lecture presented at Institute of Food Technologists Meeting and Food Expo, New Orleans, LA, June 5, 2019.

Hasek, Like Y., Robert J. Phillips, Genyi Zhang, Kimberly P. Kinzig, et al. "Dietary Slowly Digestible Starch Triggers the Gut-Brain Axis in Obese Rats with Accompanied Reduced Food Intake." *Molecular Nutrition & Food Research* 62, no. 5 (February 22, 2018): 1700117, doi:10.1002/mnfr.201700117.

Hätönen, Katja A., Jarmo Virtamo, Johan G. Eriksson, Harri K. Sinkko, et al. "Protein and Fat Modify the Glycaemic and Insulinaemic Responses to a Mashed Potato–Based Meal." *British Journal of Nutrition* 106, no. 2 (July 28, 2011): 248–53.

Heaton, K. W., S. N. Marcus, P. M. Emmett, and C. H. Bolton. "Particle Size of Wheat, Maize, and Oat Test Meals: Effects on Plasma Glucose and Insulin Responses and on the Rate of Starch Digestion In Vitro." *American Journal of Clinical Nutrition* 47, no. 4 (April 1988): 675–82.

Holm, Jörgen, Barbro Hagander, Inger Björck, Ann-Charlotte Eliasson, and Ingmar Lundquist. "The Effect of Various Thermal Processes on the Glycemic Response to Whole Grain Wheat Products in Humans and Rats." *Journal of Nutrition* 119, no. 11 (November 1, 1989): 1631–38, doi: 10.1093/jn/119.11.1631.

Hudson, Geoffrey, and Hans Englyst. "Carbohydrates in Food Tables." *Food Chemistry* 57, no. 1 (1996): 37.

Juntunen, Katri S., Leo K. Niskanen, Kirsi H. Liukkonen, Kaisa S. Poutanen, et al. "Postprandial Glucose, Insulin, and Incretin Responses to Grain Products in Healthy Subjects." *American Journal of Clinical Nutrition* 75, no. 2 (February 2002): 254–62.

Kendall, Cyril W. C., Livia S. A. Augustin, Azadeh Emam, Andrea R. Josse, et al. "The Glycemic Index: Methodology and Use." *Nutritional Management of Diabetes Mellitus and Dysmetabolic Syndrome* (2006): 43–56, doi:10.1159/000094405.

Larsen, Philip J. "Mechanisms behind GLP-1 Induced Weight Loss." *British Journal of Diabetes & Vascular Disease* 8, suppl. 2 (November 2008): S34–S41, doi:10.1177/1474651408100525.

Lee, Julie Anne, Geoffrey Soutar, and Jordan Louviere. "The Best–Worst Scaling Approach: An Alternative to Schwartz's Values Survey." *Journal of Personality Assessment* 90, no. 4 (June 26, 2008): 335–47, https://doi.org/10.1080/00223890802107925.

Little, Tanya J., Selena Doran, James H. Meyer, Andre J. P. M. Smout, et al. "The Release of GLP-1 and Ghrelin, but Not GIP and CCK, by Glucose Is Dependent upon the Length of Small Intestine Exposed." *American Journal of Physiology-Endocrinology and Metabolism* 291, no. 3 (September 2006): E647–E655, doi:10.1152/ajpendo.00099.2006.

Madhusudhan, Basavaraj, and Rudrapatnam N. Tharanathan. "Legume and Cereal Starches: Why Differences in Digestibility? Part II. Isolation and Characterization of Starches from Rice (*O. sativa*) and Ragi (Finger Millet, *E. coracana*)." *Carbohydrate Polymers* 28, no. 2 (January 1995): 153–58, doi:10.1016/0144-8617(95)00108-5.

Mir, Shabir Ahmad, Annamalai Manickavasagan, and Manzoor Ahmad Shah. *Whole Grains: Processing, Product Development, and Nutritional Aspects*. Boca Raton, FL: CRC Press, 2019.

Philippou, Elena. *The Glycemic Index*. Boca Raton, FL: CRC Press, 2017.

Pi-Sunyer, F. X. "Glycemic Index and Disease." *American Journal of Clinical Nutrition* 76, no. 1 (July 2002): 290S–298S.

Robertson, Denise. "Resistant Starches and Cardiometabolic Risk." Lecture presented at Nutrition Society Winter Conference 2018: Optimal Diet and Lifestyle Strategies for the Management of Cardio-Metabolic Risk, London, UK, December 5, 2018.

Seal, Chris J., Mark E. Daly, Lois C. Thomas, Wendy Bal, et al. "Postprandial Carbohydrate Metabolism in Healthy Subjects and Those with Type 2 Diabetes Fed Starches with Slow and Rapid Hydrolysis Rates Determined

In Vitro." *British Journal of Nutrition* 90, no. 5 (November 2003): 853–64, doi:10.1079/bjn2003972.

Singh, Jaspreet, Thilo Berg, Allan Hardacre, and Mike J. Boland. "Cotyledon Cell Structure and *In Vitro* Starch Digestion in Navy Beans." In *Food Structures, Digestion and Health*, ed. Mike Boland, Matt Golding, and Harjinder Singh, 223–42. San Diego, CA: Elsevier Science, 2014.

University of Sydney. "GI Foods: Bagel, White Bread." October 18, 2019, www.glycemicindex.com/foodSearch.php?num=571&ak=detail.

Unwin, David, David Haslam, and Geoffrey Livesey. "It Is the Glycemic Response to, Not the Carbohydrate Content of Food That Matters in Diabetes and Obesity: The Glycemic Index Revisited." *Journal of Insulin Resistance* 1, no. 1 (August 19, 2016), https://doi.org/10.4102/jir.v1i1.8.

Wachters-Hagedoorn, Renate E., Marion G. Priebe, Janneke A. J. Heimweg, A. Marius Heiner, et al. "The Rate of Intestinal Glucose Absorption Is Correlated with Plasma Glucose-Dependent Insulinotropic Polypeptide Concentrations in Healthy Men." *Journal of Nutrition* 136, no. 6 (June 1, 2006): 1511–16, doi:10.1093/jn/136.6.1511.

Wolever, T. M. S. "Glycemic Index Claims on Food Labels: Review of Health Canada's Evaluation." *European Journal of Clinical Nutrition* 67, no. 12 (December 2013): 1229–33.

———. "Is Glycaemic Index (GI) a Valid Measure of Carbohydrate Quality?" *European Journal of Clinical Nutrition* 67, no. 5 (May 2013): 522–31.

Woodward, A. D., P. R. Regmi, M. G. Gänzle, T. A. T. G. van Kempen, and R. T. Zijlstra. "Slowly Digestible Starch Influences mRNA Abundance of Glucose and Short-Chain Fatty Acid Transporters in the Porcine Distal Intestinal Tract." *Journal of Animal Science* 90, suppl. no. 4 (December 1, 2012): 80–82, doi:10.2527/jas.53877.

Zeller, Jonathan. "Bagelology." NYC The Official Guide Web Site, June 17, 2014, https://www.nycgo.com/articles/bagelology-scientific-study-of-nyc-bagels-slideshow.

Zhang, Genyi, and Bruce R. Hamaker. "The Nutritional Property of Endosperm Starch and Its Contribution to the Health Benefits of Whole

Grain Foods." *Critical Reviews in Food Science and Nutrition* 57, no. 18 (February 6, 2016): 3807–17, doi:10.1080/10408398.2015.1130685.

———. "Slowly Digestible Starch: Concept, Mechanism, and Proposed Extended Glycemic Index." *Critical Reviews in Food Science and Nutrition* 49, no. 10 (December 2, 2009): 852–67, doi:10.1080/1040839090337 2466.

Zhang, Genyi, Like Y. Hasek, Byung-Hoo Lee, and Bruce R. Hamaker. "Gut Feedback Mechanisms and Food Intake: A Physiological Approach to Slow Carbohydrate Bioavailability." *Food & Function* 6, no. 4 (2015): 1072–89, doi:10.1039/c4fo00803k.

Zhang, Genyi, Maghaydah Sofyan, and Bruce R. Hamaker. "Slowly Digestible State of Starch: Mechanism of Slow Digestion Property of Gelatinized Maize Starch." *Journal of Agricultural and Food Chemistry* 56, no. 12 (June 2008): 4695–702, doi:10.1021/jf072823e.

Interviews and Correspondence with the Author

Aronne, Louis J. (Dec. 2006)

Gardner, Christopher (Nov. 2018)

Hamaker, Bruce (Oct. 2018, June 2019)

Jenkins, David (June 2019)

Wolever, Thomas (Oct. 2018)

Notes

69   **This so-called ultragrain:** Ardent Mills, "Ultragrain Whole Wheat Flours."

71   **measuring insulin levels:** Eades, "Incretins."

71   **twenty-three teaspoons of sugar:** This calculation is based on: 1. A bagel weight of 184 grams (Zeller, "Bagelology"). 2. Ninety-two grams of bagel carbohydrate (50 grams of carbohydrate per 100 grams/ bagel [Fatsecret.com]). 3. A bagel glycemic index of 69 (University of Sydney). 4. A glycemic load of 63.48 in a 184-gram bagel (author's calculation using Unwin et al.'s methodology). 5. A glycemic load of 2.73 in a teaspoon of sugar (ibid.). For methodology see Unwin et al., "It Is the Glycemic Response."

Chapter 18: Highly processed carbs wreak havoc on our bodies

Sources
Works Referenced

Flatt, P. R. "Dorothy Hodgkin Lecture 2008 Gastric Inhibitory Polypeptide (GIP) Revisited: A New Therapeutic Target for Obesity-Diabetes?" *Diabetic Medicine* 25, no. 7 (July 4, 2008): 759–64.

Holst, J. J. "On the Physiology of GIP and GLP-1." *Hormone and Metabolic Research* 36, no. 11/12 (2004): 747–54.

Isken, Frank, Andreas F. H. Pfeiffer, Rubén Nogueiras, Martin A. Osterhoff, et al. "Deficiency of Glucose-Dependent Insulinotropic Polypeptide Receptor Prevents Ovariectomy-Induced Obesity in Mice." *American Journal of Physiology-Endocrinology and Metabolism* 295, no. 2 (August 1, 2008): 350–55.

Isken, F., M. Weickert, M. Tschöp, R. Nogueiras, et al. "Metabolic Effects of Diets Differing in Glycaemic Index Depend on Age and Endogenous Glucose-Dependent Insulinotrophic Polypeptide in Mice." *Diabetologia* 52, no. 10 (October 2009): 2159–68.

Jomori, Takahito, Yutaka Seino, Nobuhiro Ban, Kinsuke Tsuda, et al. "Inhibition of Gastric Inhibitory Polypeptide Signaling Prevents Obesity." *Nature Medicine* 8, no. 7 (July 2002): 738–42.

Nauck, Michael A., and Juris J. Meier. "The Incretin Effect in Healthy Individuals and Those with Type 2 Diabetes: Physiology, Pathophysiology, and Response to Therapeutic Interventions." *Lancet Diabetes & Endocrinology* 4, no. 6 (2016): 525–36.

Pfeiffer, Andreas F. H., and Farnaz Keyhani-Nejad. "High Glycemic Index Metabolic Damage: A Pivotal Role of GIP and GLP-1." *Trends in Endocrinology & Metabolism* 29, no. 5 (May 2018): 289–99.

Rudovich, Natalia, Simone Kaiser, Stefan Engeli, Martin Osterhoff, et al. "GIP Receptor mRNA Expression in Different Fat Tissue Depots in Postmenopausal Non-Diabetic Women." *Regulatory Peptides* 142, no. 3 (2007): 138–45.

Song, Mingyang, Teresa T. Fung, Frank B. Hu, Walter C. Willett, et al. "Association of Animal and Plant Protein Intake with All-Cause and

Cause-Specific Mortality." *JAMA Internal Medicine* 176, no. 10 (October 1, 2016): 1453–63, doi:10.1001/jamainternmed.2016.4182.

Interviews and Correspondence with the Author

Civille, Gail Vance (Nov. 2018, June 2019)

Chapter 19: Where we digest carbs determines how our hunger is satisfied

Sources
Works Referenced

Anderberg, Rozita H., Christine Anefors, Filip Bergquist, Hans Nissbrandt, and Karolina P. Skibicka. "Dopamine Signaling in the Amygdala, Increased by Food Ingestion and GLP-1, Regulates Feeding Behavior." *Physiology & Behavior* 136 (September 2014): 135–44, doi:10.1016/j.physbeh.2014.02.026.

Bagger, Jonatan I., Filip K. Knop, Asger Lund, Henrik Vestergaard, et al. "Impaired Regulation of the Incretin Effect in Patients with Type 2 Diabetes." *Journal of Clinical Endocrinology & Metabolism* 96, no. 3 (March 1, 2011): 737–45.

Campbell, Keith R., Michael E. Cobble, and Timothy S. Rei. "Pathophysiology of Type 2 Diabetes Mellitus: Potential Role of Incretin-Based Therapies." *Journal of Family Practice* 59, no. 9 (September 2010): S5–S9.

Dorton, Hilary M., Shan Luo, John R. Monterosso, and Kathleen A. Page. "Influences of Dietary Added Sugar Consumption on Striatal Food-Cue Reactivity and Postprandial GLP-1 Response." *Frontiers in Psychiatry* 8 (January 4, 2018), doi:10.3389/fpsyt.2017.00297.

Freeman, Jeffrey S. "Role of the Incretin Pathway in the Pathogenesis of Type 2 Diabetes Mellitus." *Cleveland Clinic Journal of Medicine* 76, no. 5 (December 2009): S12–S19.

Fujioka, Ken. "Pathophysiology of Type 2 Diabetes and the Role of Incretin Hormones and Beta-Cell Dysfunction." *Journal of the American Academy of PAs* 20, no. 12 (December 2007): 3–8.

Holst, Jens Juul, Tina Vilsbøll, and Carolyn F. Deacon. "The Incretin System and Its Role in Type 2 Diabetes Mellitus." *Molecular and Cellular Endocrinology* 297, no. 1 (January 2009): 127–36.

Jerlhag, E. "Effects of Ghrelin, Glp-1 and Amylin on Alcohol and Drug Reward." Lecture presented at the 26th Annual Meeting of the Society for the Study of Ingestive Behavior, Bonita Springs, FL, July 17–21, 2018.

Keyhani-Nejad, Farnaz, Margrit Kemper, Rita Schueler, Olga Pivovarova, et al. "Effects of Palatinose and Sucrose Intake on Glucose Metabolism and Incretin Secretion in Subjects with Type 2 Diabetes." *Diabetes Care* 39, no. 3 (March 2016): 38–39.

Leon, R. M., D. J. Reiner, L. M. Stein, B. C. De Jonghe, and M. R. Hayes. "Serotonergic Modulation of Central Glucagon-Like Peptide-1 Neurons Regulates Energy Balance and Malaise." Lecture presented at the 26th Annual Meeting of the Society for the Study of Ingestive Behavior, Bonita Springs, FL, July 17–21, 2018.

Mari, Andrea, Jonatan I. Bagger, Ele Ferrannini, Jens J. Holst, et al. "Mechanisms of the Incretin Effect in Subjects with Normal Glucose Tolerance and Patients with Type 2 Diabetes." *PLOS One* 8, no. 9 (September 3, 2013), https://doi.org/10.1371/journal.pone.0073154.

Meier, Juris J. "The Contribution of Incretin Hormones to the Pathogenesis of Type 2 Diabetes." *Best Practice & Research: Clinical Endocrinology & Metabolism* 23, no. 4 (August 2009): 433–41.

Meier, Juris J., and Michael A. Nauck. "Incretins and the Development of Type 2 Diabetes." *Current Diabetes Reports* 6, no. 3 (May 2006): 194–201.

Mossello, Enrico, Elena Ballini, Marta Boncinelli, Matteo Monami, et al. "Glucagon-Like Peptide-1, Diabetes, and Cognitive Decline: Possible Pathophysiological Links and Therapeutic Opportunities." *Experimental Diabetes Research* (2011), http://dx.doi.org/10.1155/2011/281674.

Mozaffarian, Dariush. "Starch Sugar and Metabolic Health (From Research to Practice)." Lecture presented at the American Society of Nutrition Conference, Baltimore, MD, June 8–11, 2019.

Nauck, Michael A., and Juris J. Meier. "The Incretin Effect in Healthy Individuals and Those with Type 2 Diabetes: Physiology, Pathophysiology, and Response to Therapeutic Interventions." *Lancet Diabetes & Endocrinology* 4, no. 6 (June 1, 2016): P525–P536.

Nauck, M. A., I. Vardarli, C. F. Deacon, J. J. Holst, and J. J. Meier. "Secretion of Glucagon-Like Peptide-1 (GLP-1) in Type 2 Diabetes: What Is Up, What Is Down?" *Diabetologia* 54, no. 1 (January 2011): 10–18.

Opinto, Giuseppina, Annalisa Natalicchio, and Piero Marchetti. "Physiology of Incretins and Loss of Incretin Effect in Type 2 Diabetes and Obesity." *Archives of Physiology and Biochemistry* 119, no. 4 (2013): 170–78.

Parvaresh Rizi, Ehsan, Tze Ping Loh, Sonia Baig, Vanna Chhay, et al. "A High Carbohydrate, but Not Fat or Protein Meal Attenuates Postprandial Ghrelin, PYY, and GLP-1 Responses in Chinese Men." Ed. François Blachier. *PLOS One* 13, no. 1 (January 31, 2018): e0191609, doi:10.1371/journal.pone.0191609.

Pfeiffer, Andreas F. H., and Farnaz Keyhani-Nejad. "High Glycemic Index Metabolic Damage: A Pivotal Role of GIP and GLP-1." *Trends in Endocrinology & Metabolism* 29, no. 5 (May 2018): 289–99, doi:10.1016/j.tem.2018.03.003.

Roitman, M. F. "Peripheral Hormones Tune Phasic Dopamine Responses Evoked by Nutritive and Drug Rewards." Lecture presented at the 26th Annual Meeting of the Society for the Study of Ingestive Behavior, Bonita Springs, FL, July 17–21, 2018.

Schmidt, H. D. "Can Glp-1 Receptor Antagonists Be Re-Purposed for Cocaine Addiction?" Lecture presented at the 26th Annual Meeting of the Society for the Study of Ingestive Behavior, Bonita Springs, FL, July 17–21, 2018.

Sclafani, Anthony, and Karen Ackroff. "Flavor Preferences Conditioned by Nutritive and Non-Nutritive Sweeteners in Mice." *Physiology & Behavior* 173 (2016): 188–99.

Sclafani, Anthony, Steven Zukerman, and Karen Ackroff. "Postoral Glucose Sensing, Not Caloric Content, Determines Sugar Reward in C57BL/6J Mice." *Chemical Senses* 40, no. 4 (May 2015): 245–58.

Ten Kulve, Jennifer S., Dick J. Veltman, Liselotte van Bloemendaal, Frederik Barkhof, et al. "Endogenous GLP-1 Mediates Postprandial Reductions in Activation in Central Reward and Satiety Areas in Patients with Type 2 Diabetes." *Diabetologia* 58, no. 12 (September 18, 2015): 2688–98, doi:10.1007/s00125-015-3754-x.

Terrill, S. J., M. K. Holt, S. Trapp, and D. L. Williams. "Endogenous Glp-1 in Lateral Septum Promotes Satiety and Suppresses Motivation for Food in Mice." Lecture presented at the 26th Annual Meeting of the

Notes

Society for the Study of Ingestive Behavior, Bonita Springs, FL, July 17–21, 2018.

Urbano, Francesco, Agnese Filippello, Antonino Di Pino, Davide Barbagallo, et al. "Altered Expression of Uncoupling Protein 2 in GLP-1-Producing Cells after Chronic High Glucose Exposure: Implications for the Pathogenesis of Diabetes Mellitus." *American Journal of Physiology* 310, no. 7 (April 2016): C558–C567.

Vilsbøll, Tina. "On the Role of the Incretin Hormones GIP and GLP-1 in the Pathogenesis of Type 2 Diabetes Mellitus." *Danish Medical Bulletin* 51, no. 4 (December 2004): 364–70.

Vilsbøll, T., and J. J. Holst. "Incretins, Insulin Secretion, and Type 2 Diabetes Mellitus." *Diabetologia* 47, no. 3 (March 2004): 357–66.

Vilsbøll, T., and F. K. Knop. "Effect of Incretin Hormones GIP and GLP-1 for the Pathogenesis of Type 2 Diabetes Mellitus." *Ugeskr Laeger* 169 (May 2007): 2101–5.

Wachters-Hagedoorn, Renate E., Marion G. Priebe, Janneke A. J. Heimweg, A. Marius Heiner, et al. "The Rate of Intestinal Glucose Absorption Is Correlated with Plasma Glucose-Dependent Insulinotropic Polypeptide Concentrations in Healthy Men." *Journal of Nutrition* 136, no. 6 (June 1, 2006): 1511–16, doi:10.1093/jn/136.6.1511.

Woerle, Hans Juergen, Lucianno Carneiro, Ayman Derani, Burkhard Göke, and Jörg Schirra. "The Role of Endogenous Incretin Secretion as Amplifier of Glucose-Stimulated Insulin Secretion in Healthy Subjects and Patients with Type 2 Diabetes." *Diabetes* 61, no. 9 (September 2012): 2349–58.

Interviews and Correspondence with the Author

Gribble, Fiona (May 2018)

Mozaffarian, Dariush (May 2019)

Sclafani, Anthony (May 2019)

Notes

77 **In another body of research:** Keyhani-Nejad et al., "Effects of Palatinose and Sucrose Intake."

78   **Pfeiffer and Keyhani have suggested:** Pfeiffer and Keyhani-Nejad, "High Glycemic Index Metabolic Damage."

Chapter 20: Highly processed food triggers speed eating

Sources
Works Referenced

Andrade, Chittaranjan. "Ultraprocessed Food and Cardiovascular Risk: Estimating the Number Needed to Harm in an Unfamiliar Situation." *Indian Journal of Psychological Medicine* 41, no. 5 (September 1, 2019): 501–2.

Asquith, Thomas Northrup, Brandi Rene Cole, Yonas Gisaw, Oiki Syliva Lai, and Maria Dolores Martines-Serna Villagran. Potato-based snacks and methods for preparing them. European Patent EP1043940, filed December 30, 1998, and issued July 8, 1999.

de Graaf, C., and F. J. Kok. "Slow Food, Fast Food, and the Control of Food Intake." *Nature Reviews Endocrinology* 6, no. 5 (2010): 290–93.

Ferriday, Danielle, Matthew L. Bosworth, Nicolas Godinot, Nathalie Martin, et al. "Variation in the Oral Processing of Everyday Meals Is Associated with Fullness and Meal Size: A Potential Nudge to Reduce Energy Intake?" *Nutrients* 8, no. 5 (May 21, 2016): 315.

Forde, C. G., C. Leong, E. Chia-Ming, and K. McCrickerd. "Fast or Slow-Foods? Describing Natural Variations in Oral Processing Characteristics across a Wide Range of Asian Foods." *Food & Function* 8, no. 2 (February 22, 2017): 595–606.

Forde, C. G., N. van Kuijk, T. Thaler, C. de Graaf, and N. Martin. "Oral Processing Characteristics of Solid Savoury Meal Components, and Relationship with Food Composition, Sensory Attributes, and Expected Satiation." *Appetite* 60, no. 1 (January 1, 2013): 208–19.

Gage, Dennis Roy, Steven Richard Cammarn, Richard Worthington Lodge, and Vincent York-Leung Wong. Extrusion cooked snack chips. European Patent 0287158A2, filed April 7, 1988, withdrawn.

Gage, Dennis R., Richard W. Lodge, Stephen R. Cammarn, and Vincent Y. Wong. Process for cooking extrusion cooked snack chips. U.S. Patent 5,147,675, filed September 18, 1991, and issued September 15, 1992.

Hall, Kevin D. "Carbs, Calories, or Quality? What Matters Most for Weight Control." Lecture presented at the 6th Canadian Obesity Summit, Ottawa, ON, April 23–26, 2019.

———. "Ultra-Processed Diets Cause Excess Calorie Intake and Weight Gain: An Inpatient Randomized Controlled Trial of Ad Libitum Food Intake." Lecture presented at Nutrition 2019, Baltimore, MD, June 8–11, 2019.

Hall, Kevin D., Alexis Ayuketah, Robert Brychta, Hongyi Cai, et al. "Ultra-Processed Diets Cause Excess Calorie Intake and Weight Gain: An Inpatient Randomized Controlled Trial of Ad Libitum Food Intake." *Cell Metabolism* 30, no. 1 (July 2, 2019): 67–77.

Lee, William Edwards, III, Robert Lee White, James Martein Bangel, and David Joseph Bruno Jr. (Applicant: The Procter and Gamble Company). Process for making a corn chip with potato chip texture. European Patent Application 85202059.3, filed December 12, 1985, application published July 2, 1986.

Marrón-Ponce, Joaquín A., Mario Flores, Gustavo Cediel, Carlos Augusto Monteiro, and Carolina Batis. "Associations between Consumption of Ultra-Processed Foods and Intake of Nutrients Related to Chronic Non-Communicable Diseases in Mexico." *Journal of the Academy of Nutrition and Dietetics* (June 28, 2019), https://doi.org/10.1016/j.jand.2019.04.020.

Monteiro, Carlos A., Geoffrey Cannon, Renata B. Levy, Jean-Claude Moubarac, et al. "Ultra-Processed Foods: What They Are and How to Identify Them." *Public Health Nutrition* 22, no. 5 (April 2019): 936–41.

Monteiro, Carlos A., Geoffrey Cannon, Jean-Claude Moubarac, Renata B. Levy, et al. "Freshly Prepared Meals and Not Ultra-Processed Foods." *Cell Metabolism* 30, no. 1 (July 2, 2019): 5–6.

Monteiro, Carlos Augusto, Geoffrey Cannon, Jean-Claude Moubarac, Renata Bertazzi Levy, et al. "The UN Decade of Nutrition, the NOVA Food Classification, and the Trouble with Ultra-Processing." *Public Health Nutrition* 21, no. 1 (January 2018): 5–17.

Schnabel, Laure, Emmanuelle Kesse-Guyot, Benjamin Allès, Mathilde Touvier, et al. "Association between Ultraprocessed Food Consumption and Risk of Mortality among Middle-Aged Adults in France." *JAMA Internal Medicine* 179, no. 4 (April 1, 2019): 490–98.

Scrinis, Gyorgy, and Carlos Augusto Monteiro. "Ultra-Processed Foods and the Limits of Product Reformulation." *Public Health Nutrition* 21, no. 1 (January 2018): 247–52.

van den Boer, J., J. Kranendonk, A. van de Wiel, E. Feskens, et al. "Self-Reported Eating Rate Is Associated with Weight Status in a Dutch Population: A Validation Study and a Cross-Sectional Study." *International Journal of Behavioral Nutrition and Physical Activity* 14, no. 1 (2017): 121, doi:10.1186/s12966-017-0580-1.

van den Boer, Janet, Melanie Werts, Els Siebelink, Cees de Graaf, and Monica Mars. "The Availability of Slow and Fast Calories in the Dutch Diet: The Current Situation and Opportunities for Interventions." *Foods* (Basel) 6, no. 10 (October 2, 2017): 87.

Interviews and Correspondence with the Author

Hall, Kevin (Nov. 2018)

Notes

82   **Hall launched a study:** Hall et al., "Ultra-Processed Diets."

85   **question at Nutrition 2019:** Hall, "Ultra-Processed Diets."

86   **patent application to produce:** Lee et al., Process for making a corn chip with potato chip texture.

Chapter 21: Eliminating as many fast carbs as you can is essential to weight maintenance

Sources
Works Referenced

Ang, Meidjie, and Thomas Linn. "Comparison of the Effects of Slowly and Rapidly Absorbed Carbohydrates on Postprandial Glucose Metabolism in Type 2 Diabetes Mellitus Patients: A Randomized Trial." *American Journal of Clinical Nutrition* 100, no. 4 (October 2014): 1059–68.

Astrup, Arne, Jennie Brand-Miller, and Christian Bitz. *The Nordic Way: Discover the World's Most Perfect Carb-to-Protein Ratio for Preventing Weight Gain or Regain, and Lowering Your Risk of Disease.* New York: Pam Krauss / Avery, 2017.

Blackburn, G. L., B. R. Bistrian, and J. P. Flatt. "Role of a Protein-Sparing Modified Fast in a Comprehensive Weight Reduction Program." In *Recent Advances in Obesity Research*, ed. Alan Howard. London: Newman, 1975.

Bosy-Westphal, Anja, and Manfred Müller. "Impact of Carbohydrates on Weight Regain." *Current Opinion in Clinical Nutrition and Metabolic Care* 18, no. 4 (July 2015): 389–94.

Eenfeldt, Andreas. "The Ketogenic Diet." Lecture presented at Low Carb Houston, Houston, TX, October 25, 2018.

———. *Low-Carb, High-Fat Food Revolution: Advice and Recipes to Improve Your Health and Reduce Your Weight*. New York: Skyhorse, 2014.

Goss, Amy M., Laura Lee Goree, Amy C. Ellis, Paula C. Chandler-Laney, et al. "Effects of Diet Macronutrient Composition on Body Composition and Fat Distribution during Weight Maintenance and Weight Loss." *Obesity* 21, no. 6 (June 2013): 1139–42.

Johansson, Elin V., Anne C. Nilsson, Elin M. Östman, and Inger M. E. Björck. "Effects of Indigestible Carbohydrates in Barley on Glucose Metabolism, Appetite, and Voluntary Food Intake over 16 H in Healthy Adults." *Nutrition Journal* 12, no. 1 (April 11, 2013): 46, doi:10.1186/1475-2891-12-46.

Keyhani-Nejad, Farnaz, Martin Irmler, Frank Isken, Eva Wirth, et al. "Nutritional Strategy to Prevent Fatty Liver and Insulin Resistance Independent of Obesity by Reducing Glucose-Dependent Insulinotropic Polypeptide Responses in Mice." *Diabetologia* 58, no. 2 (February 2015): 374–83.

Larsen, T. M., S. Dalskov, M. van Baak, S. Jebb, et al. "The Diet, Obesity and Genes (Diogenes) Dietary Study in Eight European Countries: A Comprehensive Design for Long-Term Intervention." *Obesity Reviews* 11, no. 1 (January 2010): 76–91.

Larsen, Thomas Meinert, Stine-Mathilde Dalskov, Marleen van Baak, Susan A. Jebb, et al. "Diets with High or Low Protein Content and Glycemic Index for Weight-Loss Maintenance." *New England Journal of Medicine* 363, no. 22 (November 25, 2010): 2102–13.

Ludwig, David S. Lecture presented at the 24th Annual Winter World Congress on Anti-Aging Medicine, Las Vegas, NV, December 9–11, 2016.

Nymo, S., S. R. Coutinho, J. Jørgensen, J. F. Rehfeld, et al. "Timeline of Changes in Appetite during Weight Loss with a Ketogenic Diet." *Interna-*

tional Journal of Obesity 41, no. 8 (April 25, 2017): 1224–31, doi:10.1038
/ijo.2017.96.

Shai, Iris, Dan Schwarzfuchs, Yaakov Henkin, Danit R. Shahar, et al.,
for the Dietary Intervention Randomized Controlled Trial (DIRECT)
Group. "Weight Loss with a Low-Carbohydrate, Mediterranean, or Low-
Fat Diet." *New England Journal of Medicine* 359, no. 3 (July 17, 2008):
229–41.

Taubes, Gary. *Good Calories, Bad Calories*. New York: Anchor, 2008.

Willett, Walter, and P. J. Skerrett. *Eat, Drink, and Be Healthy: The Harvard
Medical School Guide to Healthy Eating*. New York: Simon and Schuster,
2001.

Interviews and Correspondence with the Author

Bistrian, Bruce (Nov. 2018)

Eenfeldt, Andreas (June 2019)

Sclafani, Anthony (June 2004)

Notes

88 **The first study was done:** Blackburn, Bistrian, and Flatt, "Role of a
Protein-Sparing Modified Fast." Thanks to Gary Taubes for bringing my
attention to this study.

90 **But a large-scale European study:** Larsen et al., "Diet, Obesity and
Genes."

91 **Another research project:** Shai et al., "Weight Loss."

92 **whole grains, and olive oil:** Willett and Skerrett, *Eat, Drink, and
Be Healthy*, 14, 56.

Chapter 22: Maintaining weight loss requires us to eat less over the long term

Sources
Works Referenced

Churuangsuk, Chaitong, Daniel Griffiths, Michael E. J. Lean, and Emilie
Combet. "Impacts of Carbohydrate-Restricted Diets on Micronutrient In-

takes and Status: A Systematic Review." *Obesity Reviews* 20, no. 8 (April 22, 2019), doi:10.1111/obr.12857.

Montesi, Luca, Marwan El Ghoch, Lucia Brodosi, Simona Calugi, et al. "Long-Term Weight Loss Maintenance for Obesity: A Multidisciplinary Approach." *Diabetes, Metabolic Syndrome and Obesity: Targets and Therapy* 9 (February 26, 2016): 37–46, doi:10.2147/DMSO.S89836.

National Weight Control Registry, http://nwcr.ws/default.htm (accessed November 7, 2019).

Rosenbaum, Michael. "Obesity: A Chronic Disease Long after It Is Supposedly Cured by Weight Loss." Lecture presented at the 26th Annual Meeting of the Society for the Study of Ingestive Behavior, Bonita Springs, FL, July 17–21, 2018.

———. "Set Point Theory." 2019 Obesity Medicine Summit Recording, Houston, TX, April 3–7, 2019.

Rosenbaum, Michael, Harry R. Kissileff, Laurel E. S. Mayer, Joy Hirsch, and Rudolph L. Leibel. "Energy Intake in Weight-Reduced Humans." *Brain Research* 1350 (September 2, 2010): 95–102.

Tobias, Deirdre K., Mu Chen, JoAnn E. Manson, David S. Ludwig, et al. "Effect of Low-Fat Diet Interventions versus Other Diet Interventions on Long-Term Weight Change in Adults: A Systematic Review and Meta-Analysis." *Lancet Diabetes & Endocrinology* 3, no. 12 (December 2015): 968–79, doi:10.1016/s2213-8587(15)00367-8.

Westman, Eric C., William S. Yancy, John C. Mavropoulos, Megan Marquart, and Jennifer R. McDuffie. "The Effect of a Low-Carbohydrate, Ketogenic Diet versus a Low-Glycemic Index Diet on Glycemic Control in Type 2 Diabetes Mellitus." *Nutrition & Metabolism* 5, no. 1 (December 2008), doi:10.1186/1743-7075-5-36.

Interviews and Correspondence with the Author

Rosenbaum, Michael (July 2018)

Notes

94   **seventy-four randomized controlled trials:** Aude 2004; Ballesteros-Pomar 2010; Bazzano 2014; Bradley 2009; Brehm 2003; Brehm 2005;

Brinkworth 2004; Brinkworth 2009; Cardillo 2006; Daly 2006; Dansinger 2005; Das 2007; Davis 2009; De Luis 2009; De Luis 2012; Due 2004; Due 2008; Dyson 2007; Dyson 2010; Ebbeling 2007; Elhayany 2010; Esposito 2009; Farnsworth 2003; Foster 2003; Foster 2010; Frisch 2009; Galletly 2007; Gardner 2007; Guldbrand 2012; Haufe 2011; Iqbal 2010; Keogh 2008; Klemsdal 2010; Krauss 2006; Krebs 2012; Larsen 2011; Lasker 2008; Layman 2005; Layman 2009; Lim 2009; Luscombe 2002; Luscombe 2003; Luscombe-Marsh 2005; McAuley 2005; McAuley 2006; McLaughlin 2006; McLaughlin 2007; McMillan Price 2006; Meckling 2004; Morgan 2009; Nielsen 2005; Noakes 2005; Parker 2002; Rodrí-guez-Hernandez 2011; Ruth 2013; Sacks 2009; Samaha 2003; Saslow 2017; Seshadri 2004; Shai 2008; Stern 2004; Summer 2011; Swenson 2007; Tay 2008; Thomson 2010; Truby 2006; Tsaban 2017; Tsai 2005; Volek 2009; Wal 2007; Westman 2008; Wycherley 2012; Wycherley 2016; Yancy 2004.

94   **ten of them ultimately:** Brinkworth 2009; Dansinger 2005; Davis 2009; Foster 2003; Gardner 2007; Iqbal 2010; Klemsdal 2010; McAuley 2006; Shai 2008; Stern 2004.

94   **majority of the studies:** Six of the ten studies observed that weight loss was significantly greater in the low-carb group at six months but not at one year (Klemsdal 2010; Shai 2008; Gardner 2007; McAuley 2006; Stern 2004; Foster 2003). Three studies observed the same in absolute terms, but no significance at six months (Iqbal 2010; Brinkworth 2009; Davis 2009). Dansinger (2005) did not observe a difference between diets at any time point.

95   **adaptive thermogenesis:** Rosenbaum, "Obesity."

95   **His recent research suggests:** Rosenbaum et al., "Energy Intake in Weight-Reduced Humans."

Chapter 23: Creating new habits can lessen the appeal of fast carbs

Sources
Works Referenced

Brownell, Kelly D., and Mark S. Gold. *Food and Addiction: A Comprehensive Handbook.* New York: Oxford University Press, 2012.

Coccurello, Roberto, and Mauro Maccarrone. "Hedonic Eating and the 'Delicious Circle': From Lipid-Derived Mediators to Brain Dopamine and Back." *Frontiers in Neuroscience* 12 (2018): 271, doi:10.3389/fnins.2018.00271.

Cohen, D. A., and S. H. Babey. "Contextual Influences on Eating Behaviours: Heuristic Processing and Dietary Choices." *Obesity Reviews* 13, no. 9 (May 3, 2012): 766–79, doi:10.1111/j.1467-789x.2012.01001.x.

Kahlhöfer, J., M. Lagerpusch, J. Enderle, B. Eggeling, et al. "Carbohydrate Intake and Glycemic Index Affect Substrate Oxidation during a Controlled Weight Cycle in Healthy Men." *European Journal of Clinical Nutrition* 68, no. 9 (September 2014): 1060–66.

Kessler, David. *The End of Overeating: Taking Control of the Insatiable American Appetite.* New York: Rodale, 2009.

Leigh, Sarah-Jane, and Margaret J. Morris. "The Role of Reward Circuitry and Food Addiction in the Obesity Epidemic: An Update." *Biological Psychology* 131 (January 2018): 31–42.

Lennerz, Belinda, and Jochen K. Lennerz. "Food Addiction, High-Glycemic-Index Carbohydrates, and Obesity." *Clinical Chemistry* 64, no. 1 (January 2018): 64–71.

Matsumoto, Nancy. "If Food Addiction Is Real, How Do We Treat Eating Disorders?" *Psychology Today*, April 25, 2011, https://www.psychology today.com/us/blog/eating-disorders-news/201104/if-food-addiction-is-real -how-do-we-treat-eating-disorders.

Michaud, Andréanne, Uku Vainik, Isabel Garcia-Garcia, and Alain Dagher. "Overlapping Neural Endophenotypes in Addiction and Obesity." *Frontiers in Endocrinology* 8 (2017): 127, doi:10.3389/fendo.2017.00127.

Novelle, Marta G., and Carlos Diéguez. "Food Addiction and Binge Eating: Lessons Learned from Animal Models." *Nutrients* 10, no. 1 (January 11, 2018): 71, doi:10.3390/nu10010071.

Pivarunas, Bernadette, and Bradley T. Conner. "Impulsivity and Emotion Dysregulation as Predictors of Food Addiction." *Eating Behaviors* 19 (December 2015): 9–14.

Raymond, Karren-Lee, and Geoff P. Lovell. "Food Addiction Associations with Psychological Distress among People with Type 2 Diabetes." *Journal of Diabetes and Its Complications* 30, no. 4 (2015): 651–56.

———. "Food Addiction Symptomology, Impulsivity, Mood, and Body Mass Index in People with Type Two Diabetes." *Appetite* 95 (December 1, 2015): 383–89.

Rossi, Mark A., and Garret D. Stuber. "Overlapping Brain Circuits for Homeostatic and Hedonic Feeding." *Cell Metabolism* 27, no. 1 (January 9, 2018): 42–56.

Schulte, Erica M., Sonja Yokum, Marc N. Potenza, and Ashley N. Gearhardt. "Neural Systems Implicated in Obesity as an Addictive Disorder: From Biological to Behavioral Mechanisms." *Progress in Brain Research* 223 (2016): 329–46, doi:10.1016/bs.pbr.2015.07.011.

Shriner, Richard L. "Food Addiction: Detox and Abstinence Reinterpreted?" *Experimental Gerontology* 48, no. 10 (October 2013): 1068–74.

Sinha, Rajita. "Role of Addiction and Stress Neurobiology on Food Intake and Obesity." *Biological Psychology* 131 (January 2018): 5–13.

Swarna Nantha, Yogarabindranath, Norafidza Ashiquin Abd Patah, and Mahalakshmi Ponnusamy Pillai. "Preliminary Validation of the Malay Yale Food Addiction Scale: Factor Structure and Item Analysis in an Obese Population." *Clinical Nutrition ESPEN* 16 (December 2016): 42–47, https://doi.org/10.1016/j.clnesp.2016.08.001.

Interviews and Correspondence with the Author

O'Rahilly, Stephen (Oct. 2018)

Notes

98   **use of a heuristic:** Cohen and Babey, "Contextual Influences on Eating Behaviours."

Chapter 24: Recommendation: to avoid metabolic harm, reduce or eliminate fast carbs for good

I want to acknowledge the assistance of Viswanathan Mohan, MD, PhD, president and director of the Madras Diabetes Research Foundation in Siruseri, Chennai, for focusing my attention on a number of the studies discussed in chapters 24 and 25. See in particular V. Mohan, R. Unnikrishnan, S. Shobana, M. Malavika, et al., "Are Excess Carbohydrates the Main Link to Diabetes and Its Complications in Asians?", *Indian Journal of Medical Research* 148 (2018): 531–38, and Dr. Mohan's presentation at the 2018 American Diabetes Association conference titled "Defining a Healthy Diet—Do Fats or Carbohydrates Matter More?" on June 25, 2018. I also appreciate his kindness in sharing information on rice processing practices in India.

Sources
Works Referenced

Akhoundan, Mahdieh, Zhaleh Shadman, Parisa Jandaghi, Maryam Aboeerad, et al. "The Association of Bread and Rice with Metabolic Factors in Type 2 Diabetic Patients." Ed. Stephen L. Atkin. *PLOS One* 11, no. 12 (December 22, 2016): e0167921, doi:10.1371/journal.pone.0167921.

AlEssa, Hala B., Shilpa N. Bhupathiraju, Vasanti S. Malik, Nicole M. Wedick, et al. "Carbohydrate Quality and Quantity and Risk of Type 2 Diabetes in US Women." *American Journal of Clinical Nutrition* 102, no. 6 (November 4, 2015): 1543–53, doi:10.3945/ajcn.115.116558.

Athauda, D., and T. Foltynie. "Insulin Resistance and Parkinson's Disease: A New Target for Disease Modification?" *Progress in Neurobiology* 145–146 (October–November 2016): 98–120, doi: 10.1016/j.pneurobio.2016.10.001.

Balkau, B., M. Shipley, R. J. Jarrett, K. Pyorala, et al. "High Blood Glucose Concentration Is a Risk Factor for Mortality in Middle-Aged Nondiabetic Men: 20-Year Follow-Up in the Whitehall Study, the Paris Prospective Study, and the Helsinki Policemen Study." *Diabetes Care* 21, no. 3 (March 1, 1998): 360–67, doi:10.2337/diacare.21.3.360.

Barclay, Alan W., Peter Petocz, Joanna McMillan-Price, Victoria M. Flood, et al. "Glycemic Index, Glycemic Load, and Chronic Disease Risk: A Meta-Analysis of Observational Studies." *American Journal of Clinical Nutrition* 87, no. 3 (March 1, 2008): 627–37, doi:10.1093/ajcn/87.3.627.

Bhupathiraju, Shilpa N., Deirdre K. Tobias, Vasanti S. Malik, An Pan, et al. "Glycemic Index, Glycemic Load, and Risk of Type 2 Diabetes: Results from 3 Large US Cohorts and an Updated Meta-Analysis." *American Journal of Clinical Nutrition* 100, no. 1 (July 2014): 218–32.

Coutinho, M., H. C. Gerstein, Y. Wang, and S. Yusuf. "The Relationship between Glucose and Incident Cardiovascular Events: A Metaregression Analysis of Published Data from 20 Studies of 95,783 Individuals Followed for 12.4 Years." *Diabetes Care* 22, no. 2 (February 1, 1999): 233–40, doi:10.2337/diacare.22.2.233.

De Vegt, F., J. M. Dekker, H. G. Ruhé, C. D. A. Stehouwer, et al. "Hyperglycaemia Is Associated with All-Cause and Cardiovascular Mortality in the Hoorn Population: The Hoorn Study." *Diabetologia* 42, no. 8 (July 29, 1999): 926–31, doi:10.1007/s001250051249.

Dong, Jia-Yi, Lijun Zhang, Yong-Hong Zhang, and Li-Qiang Qin. "Dietary Glycaemic Index and Glycaemic Load in Relation to the Risk of Type 2 Diabetes: A Meta-Analysis of Prospective Cohort Studies." *British Journal of Nutrition* 106, no. 11 (September 29, 2011), 1649–54, doi:10.1017/s000711451100540x.

Figlewicz, D. P., S. B. Evans, J. Murphy, M. Hoen, and D. G. Baskin. "Expression of Receptors for Insulin and Leptin in the Ventral Tegmental Area / Substantia Nigra (VTA/SN) of the Rat." *Brain Research* 964, no. 1 (February 21, 2003): 107–15, doi:10.1016/s0006-8993(02)04087-8.

Gannon, M. C., and F. Q. Nuttall. "Effect of a High-Protein, Low-Carbohydrate Diet on Blood Glucose Control in People with Type 2 Diabetes." *Diabetes* 53, no. 9 (August 26, 2004): 2375–82, doi:10.2337/diabetes.53.9.2375.

Greenwood, D. C., D. E. Threapleton, C. E. L. Evans, C. L. Cleghorn, et al. "Glycemic Index, Glycemic Load, Carbohydrates, and Type 2 Diabetes: Systematic Review and Dose-Response Meta-Analysis of Prospective Studies." *Diabetes Care* 36, no. 12 (November 21, 2013): 4166–71, doi:10.2337/dc13-0325.

Hu, Tian, Katherine T. Mills, Lu Yao, Kathryn Demanelis, et al. "Effects of Low-Carbohydrate Diets versus Low-Fat Diets on Metabolic Risk Factors: A Meta-Analysis of Randomized Controlled Clinical Trials." *American Journal of Epidemiology* 176, suppl. 7 (October 1, 2012): S44–S54, doi:10.1093/aje/kws264.

Livesey, Geoffrey, Richard Taylor, Helen F. Livesey, Anette E. Buyken, et al. "Dietary Glycemic Index and Load and the Risk of Type 2 Diabetes: Assessment of Causal Relations." *Nutrients* 11, no. 6 (June 25, 2019): 1436, doi:10.3390/nu11061436.

Notes

Lockie, S. H., and Z. B. Andrews. "The Hormonal Signature of Energy Deficit: Increasing the Value of Food Reward." *Molecular Metabolism* 2, no. 4 (August 19, 2013): 329–36, doi:10.1016/j.molmet.2013.08.003.

Ludwig, David. Lecture at the 24th Annual Winter World Congress on Anti-Aging Medicine, Las Vegas, NV, December 9–11, 2016.

Reynolds, Andrew, Jim Mann, John Cummings, Nicola Winter, et al. "Carbohydrate Quality and Human Health: A Series of Systematic Reviews and Meta-Analyses." *Lancet* 393, no. 10170 (February 2019): 434–45, doi:10.1016/s0140-6736(18)31809-9.

Sakurai, Masaru, Koshi Nakamura, Katsuyuki Miura, Toshinari Takamura, et al. "Dietary Carbohydrate Intake, Presence of Obesity, and the Incident Risk of Type 2 Diabetes in Japanese Men." *Journal of Diabetes Investigation* 7, no. 3 (October 31, 2015): 343–51, doi:10.1111/jdi.12433.

Saslow, Laura R., Charlotte Summers, James E. Aikens, and David J. Unwin. "Outcomes of a Digitally Delivered Low-Carbohydrate Type 2 Diabetes Self-Management Program: 1-Year Results of a Single-Arm Longitudinal Study." *JMIR Diabetes* 3, no. 3 (August 3, 2018): e12, doi:10.2196/diabetes.9333.

Skytte, Mads J., Amirsalar Samkani, Amy D. Petersen, Mads N. Thomsen, et al. "A Carbohydrate-Reduced High-Protein Diet Improves HbA1c and Liver Fat Content in Weight-Stable Participants with Type 2 Diabetes: A Randomised Controlled Trial." *Diabetologia* 62, no. 11 (July 23, 2019): 2066–78, doi:10.1007/s00125-019-4956-4.

Thanarajah, Sharmili Edwin, Sandra Iglesias, Bojana Kuzmanovic, Lionel Rigoux, et al. "Modulation of Midbrain Neurocircuitry by Intranasal Insulin." *Neuroimage* 194 (July 2019): 120–27.

Villegas, Raquel, Simin Liu, Yu-Tang Gao, Gong Yang, et al. "Prospective Study of Dietary Carbohydrates, Glycemic Index, Glycemic Load, and Incidence of Type 2 Diabetes Mellitus in Middle-Aged Chinese Women." *Archives of Internal Medicine* 167, no. 21 (November 26, 2007): 2310, doi:10.1001/archinte.167.21.2310.

Interviews and Correspondence with the Author

Gannon, Mary (Oct. 2019)

Ludwig, David (Nov. 2018)

Notes

104 **Recent evidence now suggests:** Thanarajah et al., "Modulation of Midbrain Neurocircuitry."

105 **Several studies link diet:** Gannon and Nuttall, "Effect of a High-Protein, Low-Carbohydrate Diet." (Graphs have been modified for readability.)

109 **In the large-scale AlEssa study:** AlEssa et al., "Carbohydrate Quality and Quantity."

110 **Research led by:** Bhupathiraju et al., "Glycemic Index."

111 **Dr. Raquel Villegas:** Villegas et al., "Prospective Study of Dietary Carbohydrates."

111 **study of Japanese factory workers:** Sakurai et al., "Dietary Carbohydrate Intake."

Chapter 25: Consumption of fast carbs may lead to metabolic syndrome

Sources
Works Referenced

Bawden, Stephen, Mary Stephenson, Yirga Falcone, Melanie Lingaya, et al. "Increased Liver Fat and Glycogen Stores after Consumption of High versus Low Glycaemic Index Food: A Randomized Crossover Study." *Diabetes, Obesity and Metabolism* 19, no. 1 (September 29, 2016): 70–77, doi:10.1111/dom.12784.

Chiasson, Jean-Louis. "Acarbose for the Prevention of Diabetes, Hypertension, and Cardiovascular Disease in Subjects with Impaired Glucose Tolerance: The Study to Prevent Non-Insulin-Dependent Diabetes Mellitus (STOP-NIDDM) Trial." *Endocrine Practice* 12, suppl. no. 1 (January 2006): 25–30.

Chiasson, Jean-Louis, Robert G. Josse, Ramon Gomis, Markolf Hanefeld, et al. "Acarbose Treatment and the Risk of Cardiovascular Disease and Hypertension in Patients with Impaired Glucose Tolerance." *JAMA* 290, no. 4 (July 23, 2003): 486–94, doi:10.1001/jama.290.4.486.

DiNicolantonio, James J., Jaikrit Bhutani, and James H. O'Keefe. "Acarbose: Safe and Effective for Lowering Postprandial Hyperglycaemia and Improving Cardiovascular Outcomes." *Open Heart* 2, no. 1 (October 2015): e000327, doi:10.1136/openhrt-2015-000327.

Goldberg, Ira J. "Triglycerides and ASCVD in Patients with Diabetes and Insulin Resistance: Evidence Connecting Them and the Most Likely Mechanisms." Lecture presented at the Endocrine's Society ENDO 2019, New Orleans, LA, March 26, 2019.

Hodson, Leanne. "The Influence of Dietary Fatty Acids on Liver Fat Content and Metabolism." Lecture presented at Nutrition Society Winter Conference 2018, London, UK, December 4, 2018.

Lonardo, Amedeo, Stefano Ballestri, Giulio Marchesini, Paul Angulo, and Paola Loria. "Nonalcoholic Fatty Liver Disease: A Precursor of the Metabolic Syndrome." *Digestive and Liver Disease* 47, no. 3 (March 2015): 181–90.

McLaughlin, Tracey, Fahim Abbasi, Hee-Sun Kim, Cynthia Lamendola, et al. "Relationship between Insulin Resistance, Weight Loss, and Coronary Heart Disease Risk in Healthy, Obese Women." *Metabolism* 50, no. 7 (July 2001): 795–800, doi:10.1053/meta.2001.24210.

Meisinger, Christa, Susanne Rospleszcz, Elke Wintermeyer, Roberto Lorbeer, et al. "Isocaloric Substitution of Dietary Carbohydrate Intake with Fat Intake and MRI-Determined Total Volumes of Visceral, Subcutaneous, and Hepatic Fat Content in Middle-Aged Adults." *Nutrients* 11, no. 5 (May 23, 2019): 1151, doi:10.3390/nu11051151.

Park, Sunmin, Jaeouk Ahn, Nam-Soo Kim, and Byung-Kook Lee. "High Carbohydrate Diets Are Positively Associated with the Risk of Metabolic Syndrome Irrespective to Fatty Acid Composition in Women: The KNHANES 2007–2014." *International Journal of Food Sciences and Nutrition* 68, no. 4 (November 8, 2016): 479–87, doi:10.1080/09637486.2016.1252318.

Petersen, K. F. "Mitochondrial Dysfunction in the Elderly: Possible Role in Insulin Resistance." *Science* 300, no. 5622 (May 16, 2003): 1140–42, doi:10.1126/science.1082889.

Radhika, Ganesan, Rob M. Van Dam, Vasudevan Sudha, Anbazhagan Ganesan, and Viswanathan Mohan. "Refined Grain Consumption and the Metabolic Syndrome in Urban Asian Indians (Chennai Urban Rural Epidemiology Study 57)." *Metabolism* 58, no. 5 (May 2009): 675–81, doi:10.1016/j.metabol.2009.01.008.

Reaven, G. M. "Banting Lecture 1988. Role of Insulin Resistance in Human Disease." *Diabetes* 37, no. 12 (December 1, 1988): 1595–607, doi: 10.2337/diabetes.37.12.1595.

———. *Clinician's Guide to Non-Insulin-Dependent Diabetes Mellitus: Pathogenesis and Treatment.* New York: Marcel Dekker, 1989.

Reaven, Gerald M., and Jerrold M. Olefsky. "Increased Plasma Glucose and Insulin Responses to High-Carbohydrate Feedings in Normal Subjects." *Journal of Clinical Endocrinology & Metabolism* 38, no. 1 (January 1974): 151–54, doi:10.1210/jcem-38-1-151.

Reklou, Andromachi, Michael Doumas, Konstantinos Imprialos, Konstantinos Stavropoulos, et al. "Reduction of Vascular Inflammation, LDL-C, or Both for the Protection from Cardiovascular Events?" *Open Cardiovascular Medicine Journal* 12 (2018): 29–40, doi:10.2174/1874192401812010029.

Schwarz, Jean-Marc, Susan M. Noworolski, Michael J. Wen, Artem Dyachenko, et al. "Effect of a High-Fructose Weight-Maintaining Diet on Lipogenesis and Liver Fat." *Journal of Clinical Endocrinology & Metabolism* 100, no. 6 (June 2015): 2434–42, doi:10.1210/jc.2014-3678.

Shulman, Gerald I. "Mechanisms of Insulin Resistance Implications for Obesity, Lipodystrophy, and Type 2 Diabetes." Banting Lecture delivered at the 78th Scientific Sessions, American Diabetes Association, Orlando, FL, June 24, 2018.

Sievenpiper, John L. "Dietary Modification in Diabetes: Carbs versus Calories." Lecture presented at 2018 American Heart Association Scientific Sessions, Chicago, IL, November 11, 2018.

———. "Health Benefits of Slowly Digestible Starches." Lecture presented at Institute of Food Technologists Meeting and Food Expo, New Orleans, LA, June 5, 2019.

Sugino, Ikumi, Koji Kuboki, Tomoko Matsumoto, Elichi Murakami, et al. "Influence of Fatty Liver on Plasma Small, Dense LDL Cholesterol in Subjects with and without Metabolic Syndrome." *Journal of Atherosclerosis and Thrombosis* 18, no. 1 (2011): 1–7.

Tay, Jeannie, Martin I. de Bock, and Elizabeth J. Mayer-Davis. "Low-Carbohydrate Diets in Type 2 Diabetes." *Lancet Diabetes & Endocrinology* 7, no. 5 (May 2019): 331–33, doi:10.1016/s2213-8587(18)30368-1.

Tay, Jeannie, Campbell H. Thompson, Natalie D. Luscombe-Marsh, Thomas P. Wycherley, et al. "Effects of an Energy-Restricted Low-Carbohydrate, High Unsaturated Fat / Low Saturated Fat Diet versus a High-Carbohydrate, Low-Fat Diet in Type 2 Diabetes: A 2-Year Randomized Clinical Trial." *Diabetes, Obesity and Metabolism* 20, no. 4 (April 2018): 858–71, doi:10.1111/dom.13164.

Tay, Jiahui. "Lifestyle Intervention Strategies for Diabetes Management." PhD dissertation, University of Adelaide, 2016.

Notes

115 **Professor Gerald Shulman:** Shulman, "Mechanisms of Insulin Resistance Implications."

Chapter 26: Fast carbs interfere with fat metabolism

Sources
Works Referenced

Ebbeling, Cara B., Henry A. Feldman, Gloria L. Klein, Julia M. W. Wong, et al. "Effects of a Low-Carbohydrate Diet on Energy Expenditure during Weight Loss Maintenance: Randomized Trial." *BMJ* 363 (November 2018): 4583, https://doi.org/10.1136/bmj.k4583.

Hall, Kevin D. "Exploring New Assessments of Energy Intake." Lecture presented at ObesityWeek presented by The Obesity Society (TOS) in partnership with the American Society for Metabolic and Bariatric Surgery (ASMBS), Nashville, TN, November 13, 2018.

———. "Macronutrients, Weight Loss, and Energy Expenditure." Lecture presented at ObesityWeek presented by The Obesity Society (TOS) in partnership with the American Society for Metabolic and Bariatric Surgery (ASMBS), Nashville, TN, November 14, 2018.

———. "A Review of the Carbohydrate-Insulin Model of Obesity." *European Journal of Clinical Nutrition* 71, no. 3 (January 11, 2017): 323–26, doi:10.1038/ejcn.2016.260.

Tay, Jeannie. "Effects of a Low-Carbohydrate Diet on Energy Expenditure during Weight Loss Maintenance: Randomized Trial." *American Journal of Clinical Nutrition* 102, no. 4 (October 2015): 780–90.

———. "Low-Carbohydrate Diets for the Metabolic Management of Adults with Type 2 Diabetes." Lecture delivered at the 78th Scientific Sessions, American Diabetes Association, Orlando, FL, June 24, 2018.

Tay, Jeannie, Campbell H. Thompson, Natalie D. Luscombe-Marsh, Thomas P. Wycherley, et al. "Effects of an Energy-Restricted Low-Carbohydrate, High Unsaturated Fat / Low Saturated Fat Diet versus a High-Carbohydrate, Low-Fat Diet in Type 2 Diabetes: A 2-Year Randomized Clinical Trial." *Diabetes Obesity and Metabolism* 20, no. 4 (April 2018): 858–71.

Interviews and Correspondence with the Author

DeBosch, Brian (Dec. 2018)

Hall, Kevin (Nov. 2018)

Ludwig, David (Nov. 2018)

Parks, Elizabeth (Nov. 2018)

Chapter 27: A vicious cycle connecting fast carbs, obesity, and diabetes traps many people who struggle with their weight

Sources
Works Referenced

Dabelea, Dana. "Towards Primordial Prevention of Diabetes in Youth." Lecture presented at Shape the Future of Diabetes, IDF Congress 2019, BEXCO, Busan, South Korea, December 3, 2019.

Ebbeling, Cara B., Henry A. Feldman, Gloria L. Klein, Julia M. W. Wong, et al. "Effects of a Low-Carbohydrate Diet on Energy Expenditure during Weight Loss Maintenance: Randomized Trial." *BMJ* (November 14, 2018): k4583, doi:10.1136/bmj.k4583.

Ishikawa, M., M. L. Pruneda, B. Adams-Huet, and P. Raskin. "Obesity-Independent Hyperinsulinemia in Nondiabetic First-Degree Relatives of Individuals with Type 2 Diabetes." *Diabetes* 47, no. 5 (May 1, 1998): 788–92, doi:10.2337/diabetes.47.5.788.

Johnson, James D. "Caloric Restriction and Insulin." Lecture presented at Endocrine Society ENDO 2019, New Orleans, LA, March 25, 2019.

Kahn, Barbara B., and Jeffrey S. Flier. "Obesity and Insulin Resistance." *Journal of Clinical Investigation* 106, no. 4 (August 15, 2000): 473–81, doi:10.1172/jci10842.

Ludwig, David. *Always Hungry? Conquer Cravings, Retrain Your Fat Cells, and Lose Weight Permanently.* New York: Grand Central Life & Style, Hachette Book Group, 2016.

Ludwig, David S., and Cara B. Ebbeling. "The Carbohydrate-Insulin Model of Obesity: Beyond 'Calories In, Calories Out.'" *JAMA Internal Medicine* 178, no. 8 (August 1, 2018): 1098–103, doi:10.1001/jamaintern med.2018.2933.

Mehran, Arya E., Nicole M. Templeman, G. Stefano Brigidi, Gareth E. Lim, et al. "Hyperinsulinemia Drives Diet-Induced Obesity Independently of Brain Insulin Production." *Cell Metabolism* 16, no. 6 (December 2012): 723–37, doi:10.1016/j.cmet.2012.10.019.

Odeleye, O. E., M. de Courten, D. J. Pettitt, and E. Ravussin. "Fasting Hyperinsulinemia Is a Predictor of Increased Body Weight Gain and Obesity in Pima Indian Children." *Diabetes* 46, no. 8 (August 1, 1997): 1341–45, doi:10.2337/diabetes.46.8.1341.

Prakash S. S. "Models That Explain the Cause of Obesity." *Indian Journal of Endocrinology and Metabolism* 22 (August 2018): 569–70, doi:10.4103 /ijem.IJEM_67_18.

Shanik, M. H., Y. Xu, J. Skrha, R. Dankner, et al. "Insulin Resistance and Hyperinsulinemia: Is Hyperinsulinemia the Cart or the Horse?" *Diabetes Care* 31, suppl. 2 (January 28, 2008): S262–268, doi:10.2337/dc08-s264.

Sigal, R. J., M. El-Hashimy, B. C. Martin, J. S. Soeldner, et al. "Acute Post-challenge Hyperinsulinemia Predicts Weight Gain: A Prospective Study." *Diabetes* 46, no. 6 (June 1, 1997): 1025–29, doi:10.2337/diab.46.6.1025.

Templeman, Nicole M. "Effects of Insulin Gene Dosage on Murine Obesity and Lifespan." PhD dissertation, University of British Columbia, 2015.

Templeman, Nicole M., Søs Skovsø, Melissa M. Page, Gareth E. Lim, and James D. Johnson. "A Causal Role for Hyperinsulinemia in Obesity." *Journal of Endocrinology* 232, no. 3 (March 2017): R173–R183, doi:10.1530/joe-16-0449.

Templeman, Nicole M., Stephane Flibotte, Jenny H. L. Chik, Sunita Sinha, et al. "Reduced Circulating Insulin Enhances Insulin Sensitivity in Old Mice and Extends Lifespan." *Cell Reports* 20, no. 2 (2017): 451–63.

Tricò, Domenico, Andrea Natali, Silva Arslanian, Andrea Mari, and Ele Ferrannini. "Identification, Pathophysiology, and Clinical Implications of Primary Insulin Hypersecretion in Nondiabetic Adults and Adolescents." *JCI Insight* 3, no. 24 (December 20, 2018), doi:10.1172/jci.insight.124912.

Interviews and Correspondence with the Author

DeFronzo, Ralph A. (Oct. 2018)

Prakash, S. S. (July 2019)

Notes

123 **not the only possible model:** Johnson, "Caloric Restriction and Insulin."

Chapter 28: We have the ability to reverse metabolic disease

Sources
Works Referenced

Sicat, Jeffrey M. "An Obesity Medicine Approach to Managing Diabetes and Weight-Related Complications." Lecture presented at the Obesity Medicine Association, Washington, DC, September 29, 2018.

Weisenberger, Jill. *Prediabetes: A Complete Guide.* Arlington, VA: American Diabetes Association, 2018.

Interviews and Correspondence with the Author

Ludwig, David (Nov. 2018)

Chapter 29: Improving metabolic health is important for preserving cognitive function, reducing the risk of certain cancers, and improving male libido

Sources
Works Referenced

Attuquayefio, Tuki N., Iris Hovens, Alex Difeliceantonio, Michael Farrugia, et al. "Effects of Intranasal Insulin on Brain Connectivity and Cognition in Overweight/Obese Adolescents," http://www.ssib.org/public /core_routines/view_abstract_no.php?show_close_window=yes&abstract no=209.

Attuquayefio, Tuki, Richard J. Stevenson, Megan J. Oaten, and Heather M. Francis. "A Four-Day Western-Style Dietary Intervention Causes Reductions in Hippocampal-Dependent Learning and Memory and Interoceptive Sensitivity." Ed. Lin Lu. *PLOS One* 12, no. 2 (February 23, 2017): e0172645, doi:10.1371/journal.pone.0172645.

Biagi, Elena, Marco Candela, Claudio Franceschi, and Patrizia Brigidi. "The Aging Gut Microbiota: New Perspectives." *Ageing Research Reviews* 10, no. 4 (2011): 428–29.

Biagi, Elena, Claudio Franceschi, Simone Rampelli, Marco Severgnini, et al. "Gut Microbiota and Extreme Longevity." *Current Biology* 26, no. 11 (2016): 1480–85.

Biagi, Elena, Lotta Nylund, Marco Candela, Rita Ostan, et al. "Through Ageing, and Beyond: Gut Microbiota and Inflammatory Status in Seniors and Centenarians." *PLOS One* 5, no. 5 (2010): e10667.

Biessels, Geert Jan, Mark W. J. Strachan, Frank L. J. Visseren, L. Jaap Kappelle, and Rachel A. Whitmer. "Dementia and Cognitive Decline in Type 2 Diabetes and Prediabetic Stages: Towards Targeted Interventions," *Lancet Diabetes & Endocrinology* 2, no. 3 (March 2014): 246–55, doi:10.1016/s2213-8587(13)70088-3.

Boles, Annette, Ramesh Kandimalla, and P. Hemachandra Reddy. "Dynamics of Diabetes and Obesity: Epidemiological Perspective." *Biochimica et Biophysica Acta (BBA)—Molecular Basis of Disease* 1863, no. 5 (2017): 1026–36.

Bowers, Laura W., Emily L. Rossi, Ciara H. O'Flanagan, Linda A. de-Graffenried, and Stephen D. Hursting. "The Role of the Insulin/IGF System in Cancer: Lessons Learned from Clinical Trials and the Energy Balance-Cancer Link." *Frontiers in Endocrinology* 6 (May 15, 2015), doi:10.3389/fendo.2015.00077.

Boyt, A. A., Kevin Taddei, J. Hallmayer, E. Helmerhorst, et al. "The Effect of Insulin and Glucose on the Plasma Concentration of Alzheimer's Amyloid Precursor Protein." *Neuroscience* 95, no. 3 (1999): 727–34.

Calle, Eugenia E., Carmen Rodriguez, Kimberly Walker-Thurmond, and Michael J. Thun. "Overweight, Obesity, and Mortality from Cancer in a Prospectively Studied Cohort of U.S. Adults." *New England Journal of Medicine* 348, no. 17 (April 24, 2003): 1625–38, doi:10.1056/nejmoa021423.

Cevenini, Elisa, Daniela Monti, and Claudio Franceschi. "Inflamm-ageing." *Current Opinion in Clinical Nutrition & Metabolic Care* 16, no. 1 (2013): 14–20.

Chunchai, Titikorn, Bencharunan Samniang, Jirapas Sripetchwandee, Hiranya Pintana, et al. "Vagus Nerve Stimulation Exerts the Neuroprotective Effects in Obese-Insulin Resistant Rats, Leading to the Improvement of Cognitive Function." *Scientific Reports* 6, no. 1 (May 26, 2016), doi:10.1038/srep26866.

Collino, Sebastiano, Ivan Montoliu, François-Pierre J. Martin, Max Scherer, et al. "Metabolic Signatures of Extreme Longevity in Northern Italian Centenarians Reveal a Complex Remodeling of Lipids, Amino Acids, and Gut Microbiota Metabolism." *PLOS One* 8, no. 3 (2013): e56564.

Craft, Suzanne, Sanjay Asthana, David G. Cook, Laura D. Baker, et al. "Insulin Dose-Response Effects on Memory and Plasma Amyloid Precursor Protein in Alzheimer's Disease: Interactions with Apolipoprotein E Genotype." *Psychoneuroendocrinology* 28, no. 6 (2003): 809–22.

Crane, Paul K., Rod Walker, Rebecca A. Hubbard, Ge Li, et al. "Glucose Levels and Risk of Dementia." *New England Journal of Medicine* 369, no. 6 (2013): 540–48.

De Felice, Fernanda G. "Alzheimer's Disease and Insulin Resistance: Translating Basic Science into Clinical Applications." *Journal of Clinical Investigation* 123, no. 2 (2013): 531–39.

Eriksson, Joel, Robin Haring, Niels Grarup, Liesbeth Vandenput, et al. "Causal Relationship between Obesity and Serum Testosterone Status in Men: A Bi-Directional Mendelian Randomization Analysis." Ed. Cheng Hu. *PLOS One* 12, no. 4 (April 27, 2017): e0176277, doi:10.1371/journal.pone.0176277.

Fernandez, Ana M., and Ignacio Torres-Alemán. "The Many Faces of Insulin-Like Peptide Signaling in the Brain." *Nature Reviews Neuroscience* 13, no. 4 (2012): 225–39.

Ferreira, Laís S. S., Caroline S. Fernandes, Marcelo N. N. Vieira, and Fernanda G. De Felice. "Insulin Resistance in Alzheimer's Disease." *Frontiers in Neuroscience* 12 (November 2018): 830, https://doi.org/10.3389/fnins.2018.00830.

Ferroni, P., S. Riondino, A. Laudisi, I. Portarena, et al. "Pretreatment Insulin Levels as a Prognostic Factor for Breast Cancer Progression." *Oncologist* 21, no. 9 (July 7, 2016): 1041–49, doi:10.1634/theoncologist.2015-0462.

Franceschi, Claudio, and Judith Campisi. "Chronic Inflammation (Inflammaging) and Its Potential Contribution to Age-Associated Diseases." *Journals of Gerontology Series A: Biomedical Sciences and Medical Sciences* 69, suppl. 1 (2014): S4–S9.

Franceschi, Claudio, Paolo Garagnani, Paolo Parini, Cristina Giuliani, and Aurelia Santoro. "Inflammaging: A New Immune-Metabolic Viewpoint for Age-Related Diseases." *Nature Reviews Endocrinology* 14, no. 10 (2018): 576–90.

Franceschi, Claudio, Paolo Garagnani, Giovanni Vitale, Miriam Capri, and Stefano Salvioli. "Inflammaging and 'Garb-aging.'" *Trends in Endocrinology & Metabolism* 28, no. 3 (2017): 199–212.

Fulop, Tamas, Jacek M. Witkowski, Fabiola Olivieri, and Anis Larbi. "The Integration of Inflammaging in Age-Related Diseases." *Seminars in Immunology* 40 (2018): 17–35, https://doi.org/10.1016/j.smim.2018.09.003.

Giovannucci, Edward L. "Diet, Physical Activity, Metabolic Health, and Cancer Prevention." Lecture presented at American Association for Cancer Research Annual Meeting, Atlanta, GA, March 29–April 3, 2019.

Goodwin, P. J. "Fasting Insulin and Outcome in Early-Stage Breast Cancer: Results of a Prospective Cohort Study." *Journal of Clinical Oncology* 20, no. 1 (January 1, 2002): 42–51, doi:10.1200/jco.20.1.42.

Gregor, Margaret F., and Gökhan S. Hotamisligil. "Inflammatory Mechanisms in Obesity." *Annual Review of Immunology* 29 (2011): 415–445.

Groussin, M., F. Mazel, J. G. Sanders, C. S. Smillie, et al. "Unraveling the Processes Shaping Mammalian Gut Microbiomes over Evolutionary Time." *Nature Communications* 8 (February 23, 2017): 14319, doi:10.1038/ncomms14319.

Hammoud, Ahmad, Mark Gibson, Steven C. Hunt, Ted D. Adams, et al. "Effect of Roux-En-Y Gastric Bypass Surgery on the Sex Steroids and Quality of Life in Obese Men." *Journal of Clinical Endocrinology & Metabolism* 94, no. 4 (April 2009): 1329–32, doi:10.1210/jc.2008-1598.

Ikram, M. Arfan, Guy G. O. Brusselle, Sarwa Darwish Murad, Cornelia M. van Duijn, et al. "The Rotterdam Study: 2018 Update on Objectives, Design, and Main Results." *European Journal of Epidemiology* 32, no. 9 (2017): 807–50.

Lauby-Secretan, Béatrice, Chiara Scoccianti, Dana Loomis, Yann Grosse, et al. "Body Fatness and Cancer: Viewpoint of the IARC Working Group." *New England Journal of Medicine* 375, no. 8 (August 25, 2016): 794–98, doi:10.1056/nejmsr1606602.

Lee, Yun Kyung, and Sarkis K. Mazmanian. "Has the Microbiota Played a Critical Role in the Evolution of the Adaptive Immune System?" *Science* 330, no. 6012 (2010): 1768–73.

McCaffrey, Pat. "Trials of Diabetes-Related Therapies: Mainly a Bust." ALZFORUM, November 20, 2018, https://www.alzforum.org/news/conference-coverage/trials-diabetes-related-therapies-mainly-bust.

Moeller, Andrew H., Alejandro Caro-Quintero, Deus Mjungu, Alexander V. Georgiev, et al. "Cospeciation of Gut Microbiota with Hominids." *Science* 353, no. 6297 (2016): 380–82.

Omana, Juan Javier, Ronald Tamler, Erica Strohmayer, Daniel Herron, and Subhash Kini. "Sex Hormone Levels in Men Undergoing Bariatric Surgery." *Journal of the American College of Surgeons* 209, no. 3 (September 2009): S22–S23, doi:10.1016/j.jamcollsurg.2009.06.042.

Pellitero, Silvia, Izaskun Olaizola, Antoni Alastrue, Eva Martínez, et al. "Hypogonadotropic Hypogonadism in Morbidly Obese Males Is Reversed after Bariatric Surgery." *Obesity Surgery* 22, no. 12 (August 25, 2012): 1835–42, doi:10.1007/s11695-012-0734-9.

Razay, George, Anthea Vreugdenhil, and Gordon Wilcock. "Obesity, Abdominal Obesity, and Alzheimer Disease." *Dementia and Geriatric Cognitive Disorders* 22, no. 2 (2006): 173–76.

Riederer, Peter, Amos D. Korczyn, Sameh S. Ali, Ovidiu Bajenaru, et al. "The Diabetic Brain and Cognition." *Journal of Neural Transmission* 124, no. 11 (November 2017): 1431–54, doi:10.1007/s00702-017-1763-2.

Reis, L. O., W. J. Favaro, G. C. Barreiro, L. C. De Oliveira, et al. "Erectile Dysfunction and Hormonal Imbalance in Morbidly Obese Male Is Reversed after Gastric Bypass Surgery: A Prospective Randomized Controlled Trial." *International Journal of Andrology* 33, no. 5 (August 31, 2010): 736–44, doi:10.1111/j.1365-2605.2009.01017.x.

Ruiz, Henry H., Tiffany Chi, Andrew C. Shin, Claudia Lindtner, et al. "Increased Susceptibility to Metabolic Dysregulation in a Mouse Model of Alzheimer's Disease Is Associated with Impaired Hypothalamic Insulin Signaling and Elevated BCAA Levels." *Alzheimer's and Dementia* 12, no. 8 (August 2016): 851–61, https://doi.org/10.1016/j.jalz.2016.01.008.

Saiyasit, Napatsorn, Jirapas Sripetchwandee, Nipon Chattipakorn, and Siriporn C. Chattipakorn. "Potential Roles of Neurotensin on Cognition in Conditions of Obese-Insulin Resistance." *Neuropeptides* 72 (December 2018): 12–22, doi:10.1016/j.npep.2018.09.002.

Secord, Angeles Alvarez, Vic Hasselblad, Vivian E. Von Gruenigen, Paola A. Gehrig, et al. "Body Mass Index and Mortality in Endometrial Cancer: A Systematic Review and Meta-Analysis." *Gynecologic Oncology* 140, no. 1 (January 2016): 184–90, doi:10.1016/j.ygyno.2015.10.020.

Stoeckel, Luke E., Zoe Arvanitakis, Sam Gandy, Dana Small, et al. "Complex Mechanisms Linking Neurocognitive Dysfunction to Insulin Resistance and Other Metabolic Dysfunction." *F1000Research* 5 (June 2, 2016): 353, doi:10.12688/f1000research.8300.2.

Stranahan, Alexis M., Shuai Hao, Aditi Dey, Xiaolin Yu, and Babak Baban. "Blood-Brain Barrier Breakdown Promotes Macrophage Infiltration and Cognitive Impairment in Leptin Receptor–Deficient Mice." *Journal of Cerebral Blood Flow & Metabolism* 36, no. 12 (July 20, 2016): 2108–21, doi:10.1177/0271678x16642233.

Tabung, Fred K., Li Liu, Weike Wang, Teresa T. Fung, et al. "Association of Dietary Inflammatory Potential with Colorectal Cancer Risk in

Men and Women." *JAMA Oncology* 4, no. 3 (March 1, 2018): 366–73, doi:10.1001/jamaoncol.2017.4844.

Tabung, Fred K., Weike Wang, Teresa T. Fung, Stephanie A. Smith-Warner, et al. "Association of Dietary Insulinemic Potential and Colorectal Cancer Risk in Men and Women." *American Journal of Clinical Nutrition* 108, no. 2 (June 12, 2018): 363–70, doi:10.1093/ajcn/nqy093.

Talbot, Konrad, Hoau-Yan Wang, Hala Kazi, Li-Ying Han, et al. "Demonstrated Brain Insulin Resistance in Alzheimer's Disease Patients Is Associated with IGF-1 Resistance, IRS-1 Dysregulation, and Cognitive Decline." *Journal of Clinical Investigation* 122, no. 4 (2012): 1316–38.

Tangestani Fard, Masoumeh, and Con Stough. "A Review and Hypothesized Model of the Mechanisms That Underpin the Relationship between Inflammation and Cognition in the Elderly." *Frontiers in Aging Neuroscience* 11 (March 13, 2019), doi:10.3389/fnagi.2019.00056.

Tumminia, Andrea, Federica Vinciguerra, Miriam Parisi, and Lucia Frittitta. "Type 2 Diabetes Mellitus and Alzheimer's Disease: Role of Insulin Signalling and Therapeutic Implications." *International Journal of Molecular Sciences* 19, no. 11 (October 24, 2018): 3306, doi:10.3390/ijms 19113306.

Vitale, Giovanni, Stefano Salvioli, and Claudio Franceschi. "Oxidative Stress and the Ageing Endocrine System." *Nature Reviews Endocrinology* 9, no. 4 (2013): 228–40.

Wahdan-Alaswad, Reema, Zeying Fan, Susan M. Edgerton, Bolin Liu, et al. "Glucose Promotes Breast Cancer Aggression and Reduces Metformin Efficacy." *Cell Cycle* 12, no. 24 (December 15, 2013): 3759–69, doi:10.4161/cc.26641.

Watson, G. Stennis, and Suzanne Craft. "The Role of Insulin Resistance in Age-Related Cognitive Decline and Dementia." In *Diabetes and the Brain*, ed. Geert Jan Biessels and Jose A. Luchsinger, 433–57. New York: Humana Press, 2009, doi:10.1007/978-1-60327-850-8_18.

Interviews and Correspondence with the Author

Giovannucci, Edward L. (Sept. 2019)

Mucke, Lennart (July 2019)

Willette, Auriel A. (July 2019)

Chapters 30–31:
Recommendation: reduce your LDL levels to prevent heart disease

LDL causes heart disease

Sources
Works Referenced

Bhanpuri, Nasir H., Sarah J. Hallberg, Paul T. Williams, Amy L. McKenzie, et al. "Cardiovascular Disease Risk Factor Responses to a Type 2 Diabetes Care Model Including Nutritional Ketosis Induced by Sustained Carbohydrate Restriction at 1 Year: An Open Label, Non-Randomized, Controlled Study." *Cardiovascular Diabetology* 17, no. 1 (May 2018): 56, doi:10.1186/s12933-018-0698-8.

Bittner, Vera A., and Marc S. Sabatine. "How Aggressively Do We Lower LDL-C and for Which Patients." Lecture presented at Cardiometabolic Health Congress, Boston, MA, October 26, 2018.

Cardoso, Rhanderson, Joban Vaishnav, Seth Shay Martin, and Roger S. Blumenthal. "How Low Should We Decrease LDL-Cholesterol in a Cost-Effective Manner?" *American College of Cardiology* (February 16, 2018), https://www.acc.org/latest-in-cardiology/articles/2018/02/16/09/31/how-low-should-we-decrease-ldl-cholesterol-in-a-cost-effective-manner https://www.acc.org.

Clifton, P. M., and J. B. Keogh. "A Systematic Review of the Effect of Dietary Saturated and Polyunsaturated Fat on Heart Disease." *Nutrition, Metabolism and Cardiovascular Diseases* 27, no. 12 (December 2017): 1060–80, doi:10.1016/j.numecd.2017.10.010.

Ference, Brian A., Henry N. Ginsberg, Ian Graham, Kausik K. Ray, et al. "Low-Density Lipoproteins Cause Atherosclerotic Cardiovascular Disease. 1. Evidence from Genetic, Epidemiologic, and Clinical Studies. A Consensus Statement from the European Atherosclerosis Society Consensus Panel." *European Heart Journal* 38, no. 32 (April 24, 2017): 2459–72, doi:10.1093/eurheartj/ehx144.

Ferrieres, Jean, Gaetano Maria De Ferrari, Michel P. Hermans, Moses Elisaf, et al. "Predictors of LDL-Cholesterol Target Value Attainment Differ in Acute and Chronic Coronary Heart Disease Patients: Results from DYSIS II Europe." *European Journal of Preventive Cardiology* 25, no. 18 (December 2018): 1966–76, https://doi.org/10.1177/2047487318806359.

Hunninghake, D. B., E. A. Stein, and C. A. Dujavne. "The Efficacy of Intensive Dietary Therapy Alone or Combined with Lovastatin in Outpatients with Hypercholesterolemia." *Journal of Cardiopulmonary Rehabilitation* 13, no. 6 (November 1993): 440–41, doi:10.1097/00008483-199311000-00013.

Krauss, Ronald M. "Dietary Fats vs. Carbohydrates: Impact on CVD Risk." Lecture presented at the World Congress on Insulin Resistance, Diabetes & Cardiovascular Disease, Los Angeles, CA, November 29–December 1, 2018.

Mach, François, Colin Baigent, Alberico L. Catapano, Konstantinos C. Koskinas, et al. "2019 ESC/EAS Guidelines for the Management of Dyslipidaemias: *Lipid Modification to Reduce Cardiovascular Risk*: The Task Force for the Management of Dyslipidaemias of the European Society of Cardiology (ESC) and European Atherosclerosis Society (EAS)." *European Heart Journal* ehz455 (August 2019), doi.org/10.1093/eurheartj/ehz455.

Martin, Seth S. "Statin Intensity for Primary Prevention: How Much Is Enough? More Intense." Lecture presented at the American College of Cardiology Annual Scientific Session and Expo, New Orleans, LA, March 2019.

Nasir, Khurram. "Statin Intensity for Primary Prevention: How Much Is Enough?" Lecture presented at the American College of Cardiology Annual Scientific Session and Expo, New Orleans, LA, March 2019.

Nesto, Richard. "Changing the Face of Cardiovascular Disease in Diabetes." Lecture presented at the American Association of Clinical Endocrinologists, Boston, MA, May 20, 2018.

Oppenheimer, Gerald M., and I. Daniel Benrubi. "McGovern's Senate Select Committee on Nutrition and Human Needs versus the Meat Industry on the Diet-Heart Question (1976–1977)." *American Journal of Public Health* 104 (2014): 59–69, doi.org/10.2105/AJPH.2013.301464.

Sacks, Frank M., Alice H. Lichtenstein, Jason H. Y. Wu, Lawrence J. Appel, et al. "Dietary Fats and Cardiovascular Disease: A Presidential Advisory from the American Heart Association." *Circulation* 136, no. 3 (June 2017): e1–e23.

Severson, Tracy, Penny M. Kris-Etherton, Jennifer G. Robinson, and John R. Guyton. "Roundtable Discussion: Dietary Fats in Prevention of Atherosclerotic Cardiovascular Disease." *Journal of Clinical Lipidology* 12, no. 3 (June 2018): 574–82.

Regarding the Ference, Ginsberg, et al. study cited above, please pay special attention to Table I for the Bradford Hill criteria establishing causality of low-density lipoprotein and atherosclerotic cardiovascular disease and the following references cited in that table:

Baigent, C., M. J. Landray, C. Reith, J. Emberson, et al. "The Effects of Lowering LDL Cholesterol with Simvastatin plus Ezetimibe in Patients with Chronic Kidney Disease (Study of Heart and Renal Protection): A Randomised Placebo-Controlled Trial." *Lancet* 377 (2011): 2181–92.

Benn, M., G. F. Watts, A. Tybjærg-Hansen, and B. G. Nordestgaard. "Mutations Causative of Familial Hypercholesterolaemia: Screening of 98,098 Individuals from the Copenhagen General Population Study Estimated a Prevalence of 1 in 217." *European Heart Journal* 37 (2016): 1384–94.

Boekholdt, S. M., B. J. Arsenault, S. Mora, T. R. Pedersen, et al. "Association of LDL Cholesterol, Non-HDL Cholesterol, and Apolipoprotein B Levels with Risk of Cardiovascular Events among Patients Treated with Statins: A Meta-Analysis." *JAMA* 307 (2012): 1302–9.

Buchwald, H., R. L. Varco, J. P. Matts, J. M. Long, et al. "Effect of Partial Ileal By-Pass Surgery on Mortality and Morbidity from Coronary Heart Disease in Patients with Hypercholesterolemia: Report of the Program on the Surgical Control of the Hyperlipidemias (POSCH)." *New England Journal of Medicine* 323 (1990): 946–55.

Cannon, C. P., M. A. Blazing, R. P. Giugliano, A. McCagg, et al. "Ezetimibe Added to Statin Therapy after Acute Coronary Syndromes." *New England Journal of Medicine* 372 (2015): 2387–97.

CARDIoGRAMplusC4D Consortium. "A Comprehensive 1000 Genomes-Based Genome-Wide Association Meta-Analysis of Coronary Artery Disease." *Nature Genetics* 47 (2015): 1121–30.

Cholesterol Treatment Trialists' (CTT) Collaboration, C. Baigent, L. Blackwell, J. Emberson, et al. "Efficacy and Safety of More Intensive Lowering of LDL Cholesterol: A Meta-Analysis of Data from 170,000 Participants in 26 Randomised Trials." *Lancet* 376 (2010): 1670–81.

Cohen, J. C., E. Boerwinkle, T. H. Mosley Jr., and H. H. Hobbs. "Sequence Variations in PCSK9, Low LDL, and Protection against Coronary Heart Disease." *New England Journal of Medicine* 354 (2006): 1264–72.

Collins, R., C. Reith, J. Emberson, J. Armitage, et al. "Interpretation of the Evidence for the Efficacy and Safety of Statin Therapy." *Lancet* 388 (2016): 2532–61.

Cuchel, M., E. Bruckert, H. N. Ginsberg, F. J. Raal, et al. "Homozygous Familial Hypercholesterolaemia: New Insights and Guidance for Clinicians to Improve Detection and Clinical Management. A Position Paper from the Consensus Panel on Familial Hypercholesterolaemia of the European Atherosclerosis Society." *European Heart Journal* 35 (2014): 2146–57.

Emerging Risk Factors Collaboration, E. Di Angelantonio, P. Gao, L. Pennells, et al. "Lipid-Related Markers and Cardiovascular Disease Prediction." *JAMA* 307 (2012): 2499–506.

Ference, B. A., F. Majeed, R. Penumetcha, J. M. Flack, and R. D. Brook. "Effect of Naturally Random Allocation to Lower Low-Density Lipoprotein Cholesterol on the Risk of Coronary Heart Disease Mediated by Polymorphisms in NPC1L1, HMGCR, or Both: A 2 x 2 Factorial Mendelian Randomization Study." *Journal of the American College of Cardiology* 65 (2015): 1552–61.

Ference, B. A., J. G. Robinson, R. D. Brook, A. L. Catapano, et al. "Variation in PCSK9 and HMGCR and Risk of Cardiovascular Disease and Diabetes." *New England Journal of Medicine* 375 (2016): 2144–53.

Ference, B. A., W. Yoo, I. Alesh, N. Mahajan, et al. "Effect of Long-Term Exposure to Lower Low-Density Lipoprotein Cholesterol Beginning Early in Life on the Risk of Coronary Heart Disease: A Mendelian Randomization Analysis." *Journal of the American College of Cardiology* 60 (2012): 2631–39.

Holmes, M. V., F. W. Asselbergs, T. M. Palmer, F. Drenos, et al. "Mendelian Randomization of Blood Lipids for Coronary Heart Disease." *European Heart Journal* 36 (2015): 539–50.

Khera, A. V., H. H. Won, G. M. Peloso, K. S. Lawson, et al. "Diagnostic Yield of Sequencing Familial Hypercholesterolemia Genes in Patients with Severe Hypercholesterolemia." *Journal of the American College of Cardiology* 67 (2016): 2578–89.

Lauridsen, B. K., S. Stender, R. Frikke-Schmidt, B. G. Nordestgaard, and A. Tybjærg-Hansen. "Genetic Variation in the Cholesterol Transporter NPC1L1, Ischemic Vascular Disease and Gallstone Disease." *European Heart Journal* 36 (2015): 1601–8.

Linsel-Nitschke, P., A. Götz, J. Erdmann, I. Braenne, et al. "Lifelong Reduction of LDL-Cholesterol Related to a Common Variant in the LDL-Receptor Gene Decreases the Risk of Coronary Artery Disease: A Mendelian Randomisation Study." *PLOS One* 3 (2008): e2986.

Lipid Research Clinics Program. "The Lipid Research Clinics Coronary Primary Prevention Trial Results: Reduction in the Incidence of Coronary Artery Disease." *JAMA* 251 (1984): 351–64.

Nicholls, S. J., R. Puri, T. Anderson, C. M. Ballantyne, et al. "Effect of Evolocu-mab on Progression of Coronary Disease in Statin-Treated Patients: The GLAGOV Randomized Clinical Trial." *JAMA* 316 (2016): 2373–84.

Nordestgaard, B. G., M. J. Chapman, S. E. Humphries, H. N. Ginsberg, et al. "Familial Hypercholesterolaemia Is Underdiagnosed and Undertreated in the General Population: Guidance for Clinicians to Prevent Coronary Heart Disease. Consensus Statement of the European Atherosclerosis Society." *European Heart Journal* 34 (2013): 3478–90.

Prospective Studies Collaboration, S. Lewington, G. Whitlock, R. Clarke, et al. "Blood Cholesterol and Vascular Mortality by Age, Sex, and Blood Pressure: A Meta-Analysis of Individual Data from 61 Prospective Studies with 55,000 Vascular Deaths." *Lancet* 370 (2007): 1829–39.

Raal, F. J., G. J. Pilcher, R. Waisberg, E. P. Buthelezi, et al. "Low-Density Lipoprotein Cholesterol Bulk Is the Pivotal Determinant of Atherosclerosis in Familial Hypercholesterolemia." *American Journal of Cardiology* 83 (1999): 1330–33.

Sabatine, M. S., R. P. Giugliano, A. C. Keech, N. Honarpour, et al. "Evolocumab and Clinical Outcomes in Patients with Cardiovascular Disease." *New England Journal of Medicine* 376, no. 18 (2017), doi:10.1056/NEJMoa1615664.

Sabatine, M. S., R. P. Giugliano, A. C. Keech, N. Honarpour, et al. "Rationale and Design of the Further Cardiovascular Outcomes Research with PCSK9 Inhibition in Subjects with Elevated Risk (FOURIER) Trial." *American Heart Journal* 173 (2016): 94–101.

Schmidt, H. H., S. Hill, E. V. Makariou, I. M. Feuerstein, et al. "Relationship of Cholesterol-Year Score to Severity of Calcific Atherosclerosis and Tissue Deposition in Homozygous Familial Hypercholesterolemia." *American Journal of Cardiology* 77 (1996): 575–80.

Silverman, M. G., B. A. Ference, K. Im, S. D. Wiviott, et al. "Association between Lowering LDL-C and Cardiovascular Risk Reduction among Different Therapeutic Interventions: A Systematic Review and Meta-Analysis." *JAMA* 316 (2016): 1289–97.

Wiegman, A., S. S. Gidding, G. F. Watts, M. J. Chapman, et al. "Familial Hyper-Cholesterolaemia in Children and Adolescents: Gaining Decades of Life by Optimizing Detection and Treatment." *European Heart Journal* 36 (2015): 2425–37.

Interviews and Correspondence with the Author

Ballantyne, Christie (Oct. 2018)

Ference, Brian (June 2019)

Guyton, John R. (Oct. 2018)

Kane, John (Dec. 2018.

Martin, Seth (Nov. 2018)

Matry, Manuel (Oct. 2018)

Robinson, Jennifer G. (Nov. 2018)

Temple, Robert (May 2019, Oct. 2019)

Notes

138 **"How low should you go?":** Cardoso et al., "How Low Should We Decrease LDL-Cholesterol?"

139 **levels of 112 or more**: Ferrieres et al., "Predictors."

139 **McGovern Committee recognized:** Oppenheimer and Benrubi, "McGovern's Senate Select Committee."

140 **examined a trove of studies:** Clifton and Keogh, "Systematic Review."

140 **combined data from sixty-seven studies:** Ibid.

141 **European Society of Cardiology's meetings:** Ference et al., "Low-Density Lipoproteins."

142 **patients with genetic mutations:** Ibid.

142 **involving more than two million:** Ibid.

142 **"remarkably consistent" association:** Ibid.

143 **LDL and other ApoB-containing lipoproteins:** Mach et al., "2019 ESC/EAS Guidelines."

143 **"absolutely no level of LDL":** Nesto, "Changing the Face of Cardiovascular Disease."

Chapter 32: Eating less starch reduces salt intake and lowers blood pressure

Sources
Works Referenced

Arnett, Donna K., Roger S. Blumenthal, Michelle A. Albert, Andrew B. Buroker, et al. "2019 ACC/AHA Guideline on the Primary Prevention of Cardiovascular Disease: A Report of the American College of Cardiology / American Heart Association Task Force on Clinical Practice Guidelines." *Circulation* 140, no. 11 (March 17, 2019): e596–e646.

Arnett, Donna K., Amit Khera, and Roger S. Blumenthal. "2019 ACC/ AHA Guideline on the Primary Prevention of Cardiovascular Disease: Part 1, Lifestyle and Behavioral Factors." *JAMA Cardiology* 4, no. 10 (October 1, 2019): 1043–44.

Burnier, Michel. "A Pinch of Salt: Is Low Really Good for All?" Paper presented at the European Society of Cardiology Congress 2019 together with the World Congress of Cardiology, Paris, France, August 31– September 4, 2019.

"Corrigendum to 2018 ESC/ESH Guidelines for the Management of Arterial Hypertension." *European Heart Journal* 40, no. 5 (February 1, 2019): 475, doi:10.1093/eurheartj/ehy686.

Devries, Stephen. "Interventional Cardiology Delivered with a Fork." Lecture presented at Cardiovascular Health Promotion: Contemporary

Approaches to Prevention. Live meetings presented at Heart House, Washington, DC, May 30–June 1, 2019.

Institute of Medicine. *Sodium Intake in Populations: Assessment of Evidence.* Washington, DC: National Academies Press, 2013, https://doi.org/10.17226/18311.

Whelton, Paul K. "Blood Pressure Target in Adults with Hypertension and Diabetes." Lecture presented at American Heart Association Scientific Sessions, Chicago, IL, November 10–14, 2018.

Williams, Bryan, Giuseppe Mancia, Wilko Spiering, Enrico Agabiti Rosei, et al. "2018 ESC/ESH Guidelines for the Management of Arterial Hypertension." *European Heart Journal* 39, no. 33 (August 25, 2018): 3021–104, doi:10.1093/eurheartj/ehy339.

Interviews and Correspondence with the Author

Whelton, Paul K. (Nov. 2018)

Notes

146 **don't even know:** Devries, "Cardiovascular Health Promotion."

147 **"35 percent":** Institute of Medicine, "Sodium Intake in Populations."

Chapter 33: Diet or medicine to lower LDL? Probably both.

Sources
Works Referenced

Braunwald, Eugene. "What Is the Right Age to Start Lipid Lowering Therapy?" Lecture presented at the European Society of Cardiology Congress 2019, Paris, France, August 31–September 4, 2019.

Deanfield, John. "Challenges and Models in Cardiovascular Risk Management: Start Early, Invest in Your Arteries." Lecture presented at the European Society of Cardiology Congress 2019, Paris, France, August 31–September 4, 2019.

———. "Treatment Intensity in Primary and Secondary Prevention: The Role of Precision Medicine." Lecture presented at the European Society of Cardiology Congress 2019, Paris, France, August 31–September 4, 2019.

Hallberg, Sarah. "Ketogenic Diet for CVD Prevention." Lecture presented at the American Heart Association Scientific Sessions, Chicago, IL, November 10–12, 2018.

Kastelein, John. "Beyond High-Intensity Statin: Drive LDL-C as Low as You Can—Pro." Lecture presented at the European Society of Cardiology Congress 2019, Paris, France, August 31–September 4, 2019.

———. "Insights and Innovation: Can We Alter the Course of Atherosclerotic Cardiovascular Disease?" Lecture presented at the European Society of Cardiology Congress 2019, Paris, France, August 31–September 4, 2019.

"Low-Density Lipoprotein Cholesterol and Coronary Heart Disease: Lower Is Better." *European Cardiology* 1, no. 1 (2005): 1–6, https://doi.org/10.15420/ecr.2005.1c.

Martínez-González, Miguel. "Oils, Nuts, and Sun: The Mediterranean Diet." Lecture presented at the American Heart Association Scientific Sessions, Chicago, IL, November 10–12, 2018.

Williams, Kim Allan. "Plant Power: Whole Food Plant-Based Diets." Lecture presented at the American Heart Association Scientific Sessions, Chicago, IL, November 10–12, 2018.

Yusuf, Salim. "How to Reduce Global CVD by 30 Percent by 2030: The Vision." Lecture presented at the European Society of Cardiology Congress 2019, Paris, France, August 31–September 4, 2019.

Interviews and Correspondence with the Author

Braunwald, Eugene (Sept. 2019)

Notes

148 **time to stop quibbling:** Yusuf, "How to Reduce Global CVD."

148 **a much bigger impact:** Ibid.

149 **Reducing LDL over a lifetime:** Kastelein, "Beyond High-Intensity Statin."

150 **"accumulating atherosclerosis":** Deanfield, "Challenges and Models in Cardiovascular Risk Management."

150 **"Early action":** Ibid.

Chapter 34: Recommendation: engage in daily moderate-intensity exercise to stay healthy

Sources
Works Referenced

François, Monique E., Jenna B. Gillen, and Jonathan P. Little. "Carbohydrate-Restriction with High-Intensity Interval Training: An Optimal Combination for Treating Metabolic Diseases?" *Frontiers in Nutrition* 4 (October 12, 2017), doi:10.3389/fnut.2017.00049.

Haus, Jacob. "Exercise-Enhanced Systemic Insulin Sensitivity." Lecture presented at the American Heart Association Scientific Sessions, Chicago, IL, November 10–12, 2018.

Hill, James O. "Is Exercise Necessary to Maintain a Healthy Weight?" Lecture presented at ObesityWeek presented by The Obesity Society in partnership with the American Society for Metabolic and Bariatric Surgery (ASMBS), Nashville, TN, November 13, 2018.

Interviews and Correspondence with the Author

Haus, Jacob (Nov. 2018)

Notes

152 **"increases your energy expenditure":** Hill, "Is Exercise Necessary?"

152 **"with food restriction alone":** Ibid.

152 **"fix your broken metabolism":** Ibid.

Chapter 35: Most successful diets have one thing in common: limited fast carbs

Sources
Works Referenced

Gardner, Christopher D., John F. Trepanowski, Liana C. Del Gobbo, Michelle E. Hauser, et al. "Effect of Low-Fat vs. Low-Carbohydrate Diet on 12-Month Weight Loss in Overweight Adults and the Association with

Notes

Genotype Pattern or Insulin Secretion." *JAMA* 319, no. 7 (February 20, 2018): 667–79, doi:10.1001/jama.2018.0245.

Hallberg, Sarah. "Diets from Vegan to Ketogenic: What's the Best for CV Health and for Which Patient?" Paper presented at the American Heart Association's Scientific Sessions, Chicago, IL, November 10–12, 2018.

Martínez-González, Miguel A. "Oil, Nuts, and Sun: The Mediterranean Diet." Lecture presented at the American Heart Association's Scientific Sessions, Chicago, IL, November 10–12, 2018.

Williams, Kim Allan. "Plant Power: Whole Food Plant-Based Diets." Lecture presented at the American Heart Association's Scientific Sessions, Chicago, IL, November 10–12, 2018.

Interviews and Correspondence with the Author

Gardner, Christopher (Oct. 2018)

Chapter 36: A diet emphasizing plants and slow carbs is optimal for your health

Sources
Works Referenced

Barnard, Neal D., Joshua Cohen, David J. A. Jenkins, G. Turner-McGrievy, et al. "A Low-Fat Vegan Diet and a Conventional Diabetes Diet in the Treatment of Type 2 Diabetes: A Randomized, Controlled, 74-Week Clinical Trial." *American Journal of Clinical Nutrition* 89, no. 5 (April 1, 2009): 1588S–1596S, doi:10.3945.

Barnard, N. D., J. Cohen, D. J. A. Jenkins, G. Turner-McGrievy, et al. "A Low-Fat Vegan Diet Improves Glycemic Control and Cardiovascular Risk Factors in a Randomized Clinical Trial in Individuals with Type 2 Diabetes." *Diabetes Care* 29, no. 8 (July 27, 2006): 1777–83.

Dhingra, Ravi, Philimon Gona, Byung-Ho Nam, Ralph B. D'Agostino Sr., et al. "C-Reactive Protein, Inflammatory Conditions, and Cardiovascular Disease Risk." *American Journal of Medicine* 120, no. 12 (December 2007): 1054–62, doi:10.1016/j.amjmed.2007.08.037.

Ostfeld, Robert J. "A Plant-Based Diet and Cardiovascular Health." Lecture presented at the American College of Cardiology 68th Annual Scientific Session and Expo, New Orleans, LA, March 16–18, 2019.

Oyebode, Oyinlola, Vanessa Gordon-Dseagu, Alice Walker, and Jennifer S. Mindell. "Fruit and Vegetable Consumption and All-Cause, Cancer, and CVD Mortality: Analysis of Health Survey for England Data." *Journal of Epidemiology and Community Health* 68, no. 9 (March 31, 2014): 856–62.

Satija, Ambika, Shilpa N. Bhupathiraju, Donna Spiegelman, Stephanie E. Chiuve, et al. "Healthful and Unhealthful Plant-Based Diets and the Risk of Coronary Heart Disease in U.S. Adults." *Journal of the American College of Cardiology* 70, no. 4 (July 2017): 411–22, doi:10.1016/j.jacc.2017.05.047.

———. "Plant-Based Diets and the Risk of Coronary Heart Disease in US Adults." *FASEB Journal* 31, no. 1_supplement (April 1, 2017), https://www.fasebj.org/doi/abs/10.1096/fasebj.31.1_supplement.167.4.

Wang, X., Y. Ouyang, J. Liu, M. Zhu, et al. "Fruit and Vegetable Consumption and Mortality from All Causes, Cardiovascular Disease, and Cancer: Systematic Review and Dose-Response Meta-Analysis of Prospective Cohort Studies." *BMJ* 349, (September 3, 2014): g5472. doi:https://doi.org/10.1136/bmj.g5472.

Wong, Nathan D. "How to Reduce Global CVD by 30% by 2030." Lecture presented at the European Society of Cardiology Congress 2019, Paris, France, August 31–September 4, 2019.

Notes

165 **It also lowers C-reactive protein:** Dhingra et al., "C-Reactive Protein."

165 **In a randomized control trial:** Barnard et al., "Low-Fat Vegan Diet."

165 **large-scale study:** Satija et al., "Plant-Based Diets."

165 **In a meta-analysis:** Wang et al., "Fruit and Vegetable Consumption."

Chapter 37: The pros and cons of low-carb diets

Sources
Works Referenced

Athinarayanan, Shaminie J., Rebecca N. Adams, Sarah J. Hallberg, Amy L. McKenzie, et al. "Long-Term Effects of a Novel Continuous Remote Care

Intervention Including Nutritional Ketosis for the Management of Type 2 Diabetes: A 2-Year Non-Randomized Clinical Trial." *Frontiers in Endocrinology* (June 5, 2019), https://doi.org/10.3389/fendo.2019.00348.

Atkins, Robert. *Dr. Atkins' Diet Revolution: The High-Calorie Way to Stay Thin Forever.* New York: D. McKay, 1972.

Baigent, C., L. Blackwell, J. Emberson, L. E. Holland, et al. "Efficacy and Safety of More Intensive Lowering of LDL Cholesterol: A Meta-Analysis of Data from 170,000 Participants in 26 Randomised Trials." *Lancet* 376 (2010): 1670–81.

Baigent, C., A. Keech, P. M. Kearney, L. Blackwell, et al. "Efficacy and Safety of Cholesterol-Lowering Treatment: Prospective Meta-Analysis of Data from 90,056 Participants in 14 Randomised Trials of Statins." *The Lancet* 366, no. 9493 (October 2005): 1267–78, doi:10.1016/s0140-6736(05)67394-1. (Published corrections appear in *Lancet* 366, no. 9494 [2005]: 1358; and *Lancet* 371, no. 9630 [2008]: 2084.)

Bhanpuri, Nasir H., Sarah J. Hallberg, Paul T. Williams, Amy L. McKenzie, et al. "Cardiovascular Disease Risk Factor Responses to a Type 2 Diabetes Care Model Including Nutritional Ketosis Induced by Sustained Carbohydrate Restriction at 1 Year: An Open-Label, Non-Randomized, Controlled Study." *Cardiovascular Diabetology* 17, no. 1 (May 1, 2018), doi:10.1186/s12933-018-0698-8.

Boden, Guenther, Karin Sargrad, Carol Homko, Maria Mozzoli, and T. Peter Stein. "Effect of a Low-Carbohydrate Diet on Appetite, Blood Glucose Levels, and Insulin Resistance in Obese Patients with Type 2 Diabetes." *Annals of Internal Medicine* 142, no. 6 (March 15, 2005): 403–11, doi:10.7326/0003-4819-142-6-200503150-00006.

Brouwer, Ingeborg A. "Effects of *Trans*-Fatty Acid Intake on Blood Lipids and Lipoproteins: A Systematic Review and Meta-Regression Analysis." World Health Organization, Geneva, 2016.

Cholesterol Treatment Trialists' (CTT) Collaboration, C. Baigent, L. Blackwell, J. Emberson, et al. "Efficacy and Safety of More Intensive Lowering of LDL Cholesterol: A Meta-Analysis of Data from 170,000 Participants in 26 Randomised Trials." *Lancet* 376, no. 9753 (November 2010): 1670–81, doi:10.1016/s0140-6736(10)61350-5.

Cholesterol Treatment Trialists' (CTT) Collaboration, C. Baigent, A. Keech, P. M. Kearney, et al. "Efficacy and Safety of Cholesterol-Lowering Treatment: Prospective Meta-Analysis of Data from 90,056 Participants in 14 Randomised Trials of Statins." *Lancet* 366, no. 9493 (2005): 1267–78.

Cohen, Jonathan C., Eric Boerwinkle, Thomas H. Mosley Jr., and Helen H. Hobbs. "Sequence Variations in PCSK9, Low LDL, and Protection against Coronary Heart Disease." *New England Journal of Medicine* 354, no. 12 (2006): 1264–72.

Dron, Jacqueline S., and Robert A. Hegele. "Complexity of Mechanisms among Human Proprotein Convertase Subtilisin-Kexin Type 9 Variants." *Current Opinion in Lipidology* 28, no. 2 (2017): 161–69.

Eckel, Robert H., John M. Jakicic, Jamy D. Ard, Janet M. de Jesus, et al. "2013 AHA/ACC Guideline on Lifestyle Management to Reduce Cardiovascular Risk: A Report of the American College of Cardiology / American Heart Association Task Force on Practice Guidelines." *Journal of the American College of Cardiology* 63, no. 25 Part B (2014): 2960–84. ("Correction to: 2016 ACC/AHA/HFSA Focused Update on New Pharmacological Therapy for Heart Failure: An Update of the 2013 ACCF/AHA Guideline for the Management of Heart Failure: A Report of the American College of Cardiology Foundation / American Heart Association Task Force on Clinical Practice Guidelines and the Heart Failure Society of America." *Circulation* 134, no. 13 [September 27, 2016], doi:10.1161/cir.0000000000000460.)

Emerging Risk Factors Collaboration. "Lipid-Related Markers and Cardiovascular Disease Prediction." *JAMA* 307, no. 23 (June 20, 2012): 2499–506, doi:10.1001/jama.2012.6571.

Ference, Brian A. "Causal Effect of Lipids and Lipoproteins on Atherosclerosis: Lessons from Genomic Studies." *Cardiology Clinics* 36, no. 2 (May 2018): 203–11, doi:10.1016/j.ccl.2017.12.001.

Ference, Brian A., Deepak L. Bhatt, Alberico L. Catapano, Chris J. Packard, et al. "Association of Genetic Variants Related to Combined Exposure to Lower Low-Density Lipoproteins and Lower Systolic Blood Pressure with Lifetime Risk of Cardiovascular Disease." *JAMA* 322, no. 14 (October 8, 2019): 1381N91, doi:10.1001/jama.2019.14120.

Ference, Brian A., Henry N. Ginsberg, Ian Graham, Kausik K. Ray, et al. "Low-Density Lipoproteins Cause Atherosclerotic Cardiovascular

Disease. 1. Evidence from Genetic, Epidemiologic, and Clinical Studies. A Consensus Statement from the European Atherosclerosis Society Consensus Panel." *European Heart Journal* 38, no. 32 (2017): 2459–72.

Ference, Brian A., John J. P. Kastelein, Henry N. Ginsberg, M. John Chapman, et al. "Association of Genetic Variants Related to CETP Inhibitors and Statins with Lipoprotein Levels and Cardiovascular Risk." *JAMA* 318, no. 10 (September 12, 2017): 947–56, doi:10.1001/jama.2017.11467.

Ference, Brian A., John J. P. Kastelein, Kausik K. Ray, Henry N. Ginsberg, et al. "Association of Triglyceride-Lowering LPL Variants and LDL-C-Lowering LDLR Variants with Risk of Coronary Heart Disease." *JAMA* 321, no. 4 (January 29, 2019): 364–73, doi:10.1001/jama.2018.20045.

Ference, Brian A., Faisal Majeed, Raju Penumetcha, John M. Flack, and Robert D. Brook. "Effect of Naturally Random Allocation to Lower Low-Density Lipoprotein Cholesterol on the Risk of Coronary Heart Disease Mediated by Polymorphisms in NPC1L1, HMGCR, or Both: A 2 × 2 Factorial Mendelian Randomization Study." *Journal of the American College of Cardiology* 65, no. 15 (2015): 1552–61.

Ference, Brian A., Jennifer G. Robinson, Robert D. Brook, Alberico L. Catapano, et al. "Variation in PCSK9 and HMGCR and Risk of Cardiovascular Disease and Diabetes." *New England Journal of Medicine* 375, no. 22 (2016): 2144–53.

Ference, Brian A., Wonsuk Yoo, Issa Alesh, Nitin Mahajan, et al. "Effect of Long-Term Exposure to Lower Low-Density Lipoprotein Cholesterol Beginning Early in Life on the Risk of Coronary Heart Disease." *Journal of the American College of Cardiology* 60, no. 25 (December 2012): 2631–39, doi:10.1016/j.jacc.2012.09.017.

Foscolou, A., S. Tyrovolas, A. L. Matalas, E. Magriplis, et al. "Macronutrients, Successful Aging, and Cardiometabolic Burden: A Combined Analysis of Two Epidemiological Studies." Poster presented at EuroPrevent 2019, Lisbon, Portugal, April 12, 2019.

Gibson, A. A., R. V. Seimon, C. M. Y. Lee, J. Ayre, et al. "Do Ketogenic Diets Really Suppress Appetite? A Systematic Review and Meta-Analysis." *Obesity Reviews* 16, no. 1 (November 17, 2014): 64–76, doi:10.1111/obr.12230.

Gjuladin-Hellon, Teuta, Ian G. Davies, Peter Penson, and Raziyeh Amiri Baghbadorani. "Effects of Carbohydrate-Restricted Diets on Low-Density

Lipoprotein Cholesterol Levels in Overweight and Obese Adults: A Systematic Review and Meta-Analysis." *Nutrition Reviews* 77, no. 3 (December 13, 2018): 161–80, doi:10.1093/nutrit/nuy049.

Global Lipids Genetic Consortium. "Discovery and Refinement of Loci Associated with Lipid Levels." *Nature Genetics* 45, no. 11 (October 6, 2013): 1274–83, doi:10.1038/ng.2797.

Goss, Amy M. "Diets in the News: What, When, or How Much? Ketogenic Diet." Lecture presented at ObesityWeek presented by The Obesity Society (TOS) in partnership with the American Society for Metabolic and Bariatric Surgery (ASMBS), Nashville, TN, November 13, 2018.

———. "Ketogenic Diet." Lecture presented at ObesityWeek presented by The Obesity Society (TOS) in partnership with the American Society for Metabolic and Bariatric Surgery (ASMBS), Nashville, TN, November 13, 2018.

Gower, Barbara A., Paula C. Chandler-Laney, Fernando Ovalle, Laura Lee Goree, et al. "Favourable Metabolic Effects of a Eucaloric Lower-Carbohydrate Diet in Women with PCOS." *Clinical Endocrinology* 79, no. 4 (May 20, 2013), 550–57, doi:10.1111/cen.12175.

Gower, Barbara A., and Amy M. Goss. "A Lower-Carbohydrate, Higher-Fat Diet Reduces Abdominal and Intermuscular Fat and Increases Insulin Sensitivity in Adults at Risk of Type 2 Diabetes." *Journal of Nutrition* 145, no. 1 (December 3, 2014): 177S–183S, doi:10.3945/jn.114.195065.

Hallberg, Sarah J., Amy L. McKenzie, Paul T. Williams, Nasir H. Bhanpuri, et al. "Effectiveness and Safety of a Novel Care Model for the Management of Type 2 Diabetes at 1 Year: An Open-Label, Non-Randomized, Controlled Study." *Diabetes Therapy* 9, no. 2 (February 7, 2018): 583–612, doi:10.1007/s13300-018-0373-9.

Holmes, M. V., F. W. Asselbergs, T. M. Palmer, F. Drenos, et al. "Mendelian Randomization of Blood Lipids for Coronary Heart Disease." *European Heart Journal* 36, no. 9 (March 1, 2015): 539–50, doi:10.1093/eurheartj/eht571.

Huntriss, Rosemary, Malcolm Campbell, and Carol Bedwell. "The Interpretation and Effect of a Low-Carbohydrate Diet in the Management of Type 2 Diabetes: A Systematic Review and Meta-Analysis of Randomised

Controlled Trials." *European Journal of Clinical Nutrition* 72, no. 3 (December 21, 2017): 311–25, doi:10.1038/s41430-017-0019-4.

Johnstone, Alexandra M., Graham W. Horgan, Sandra D. Murison, David M. Bremner, and Gerald E. Lobley. "Effects of a High-Protein Ketogenic Diet on Hunger, Appetite, and Weight Loss in Obese Men Feeding Ad Libitum." *American Journal of Clinical Nutrition* 87, no. 1 (January 1, 2008): 44–55, doi:10.1093/ajcn/87.1.44.

Korsmo-Haugen, Henny-Kristine, Kjetil G. Brurberg, Jim Mann, and Anne-Marie Aas. "Carbohydrate Quantity in the Dietary Management of Type 2 Diabetes: A Systematic Review and Meta-Analysis." *Diabetes, Obesity and Metabolism* 21, no. 1 (September 10, 2018): 15–27, doi:10.1111/dom.13499.

Langlois, Michel R., M. John Chapman, Christa Cobbaert, Samia Mora, et al. "Quantifying Atherogenic Lipoproteins: Current and Future Challenges in the Era of Personalized Medicine and Very Low Concentrations of LDL Cholesterol. A Consensus Statement from EAS and EFLM." *Clinical Chemistry* 64, no. 7 (2018): 1006–33.

Lewis, G. F., C. Xiao, and R. A. Hegele. "Hypertriglyceridemia in the Genomic Era: A New Paradigm." *Endocrine Reviews* 36, no. 1 (2015): 131–47.

Mach, François, Colin Baigent, Alberico L. Catapano, Konstantinos C. Koskinas, et al. "2019 ESC/EAS Guidelines for the Management of Dyslipidaemias: *Lipid Modification to Reduce Cardiovascular Risk*: The Task Force for the Management of Dyslipidaemias of the European Society of Cardiology (ESC) and European Atherosclerosis Society (EAS)." *European Heart Journal* (August 31, 2019), https://doi.org/10.1093/eurheartj/ehz455.

Mansoor, Nadia, Kathrine J. Vinknes, Marit B. Veierød, and Kjetil Retterstøl. "Effects of Low-Carbohydrate Diets v. Low-Fat Diets on Body Weight and Cardiovascular Risk Factors: A Meta-Analysis of Randomised Controlled Trials." *British Journal of Nutrition* 115, no. 3 (December 4, 2015): 466–79, doi:10.1017/s0007114515004699.

McArdle, P. D., S. M. Greenfield, S. K. Rilstone, P. Narendran, et al. "Carbohydrate Restriction for Glycaemic Control in Type 2 Diabetes: A Systematic Review and Meta-Analysis." *Diabetic Medicine* 36, no. 3 (January 3, 2019): 335–48, doi:10.1111/dme.13862.

Mensink, R. P. *Effects of Saturated Fatty Acids on Serum Lipids and Lipoproteins: A Systematic Review and Regression Analysis.* Geneva: World Health Organization, 2016.

Mozaffarian, Dariush, Tao Hao, Eric B. Rimm, Walter C. Willett, and Frank B. Hu. "Changes in Diet and Lifestyle and Long-Term Weight Gain in Women and Men." *New England Journal of Medicine* 364, no. 25 (June 23, 2011): 2392–404, doi:10.1056/nejmoa1014296.

Nikpay, Majid, Anuj Goel, Hong-Hee Won, Leanne M. Hall, et al. "A Comprehensive 1000 Genomes-Based Genome-Wide Association Meta-Analysis of Coronary Artery Disease." *Nature Genetics* 47, no. 10 (2015): 1121–30.

Phinney, Stephen. "The Safety and Efficacy of a Well-Formulated Ketogenic Diet in the Management of Type 2 Diabetes and Cardio-Metabolic Risk." Lecture presented at the Nutrition Society Winter Conference 2018, London, UK, December 4, 2018.

Sainsbury, Emma, Nathalie V. Kizirian, Stephanie R. Partridge, Timothy Gill, et al. "Effect of Dietary Carbohydrate Restriction on Glycemic Control in Adults with Diabetes: A Systematic Review and Meta-Analysis." *Diabetes Research and Clinical Practice* 139 (May 2018): 239–52, doi: 10.1016/j.diabres.2018.02.026.

Silverman, Michael G., Brian A. Ference, Kyungah Im, Stephen D. Wiviott, et al. "Association between Lowering LDL-C and Cardiovascular Risk Reduction among Different Therapeutic Interventions." *JAMA* 316, no. 12 (September 27, 2016): 1289–97, doi:10.1001/jama.2016.13985.

Snorgaard, Ole, Grith M. Poulsen, Henning K. Andersen, and Arne Astrup. "Systematic Review and Meta-Analysis of Dietary Carbohydrate Restriction in Patients with Type 2 Diabetes." *BMJ Open Diabetes Research & Care* 5, no. 1 (February 2017): e000354, doi:10.1136/bmj drc-2016-000354.

Song, Mingyang, Teresa T. Fung, Frank B. Hu, Walter C. Willett, et al. "Association of Animal and Plant Protein Intake with All-Cause and Cause-Specific Mortality." *JAMA Internal Medicine* 176, no. 10 (October 2016): 1453–63, doi:10.1001/jamainternmed.2016.4182.

Tay, Jeannie. "Low-Carbohydrate Diets for the Metabolic Management of Adults with Type 2 Diabetes." Lecture delivered at the 78th Scientific Sessions, American Diabetes Association, Orlando, FL, June 24, 2018.

Notes

Tay, Jeannie, Martin I. de Bock, and Elizabeth J. Mayer-Davis. "Low-Carbohydrate Diets in Type 2 Diabetes." *Lancet Diabetes & Endocrinology* 7, no. 5 (2019): 331–33.

Tay, Jeannie, Campbell H. Thompson, Natalie D. Luscombe-Marsh, Thomas P. Wycherley, et al. "Effects of an Energy-Restricted Low-Carbohydrate, High Unsaturated Fat / Low Saturated Fat Diet versus a High-Carbohydrate, Low-Fat Diet in Type 2 Diabetes: A 2-Year Randomized Clinical Trial." *Diabetes, Obesity, and Metabolism* 20, no. 4 (April 2018): 858–71, doi:10.111/dom./13164.

Triglyceride Coronary Disease Genetics Consortium and Emerging Risk Factors Collaboration. "Triglyceride-Mediated Pathways and Coronary Disease: Collaborative Analysis of 101 Studies." *Lancet* 375, no. 9726 (2010): 1634–39.

Van Zuuren, Esther J., Zbys Fedorowicz, Ton Kuijpers, and Hanno Pijl. "Effects of Low-Carbohydrate- Compared with Low-Fat-Diet Interventions on Metabolic Control in People with Type 2 Diabetes: A Systematic Review Including GRADE Assessments." *American Journal of Clinical Nutrition* 108, no. 2 (July 11, 2018): 300–331, doi:10.1093/ajcn/nqy096.

Varbo, Anette, Marianne Benn, Anne Tybjærg-Hansen, Anders B. Jørgensen, et al. "Remnant Cholesterol as a Causal Risk Factor for Ischemic Heart Disease." *Journal of the American College of Cardiology* 61, no. 4 (2013): 427–36.

Virta (Brittanie Volk, presenter). "Clinical Management of Carbohydrate Restriction in Type 2 Diabetes." Virta webinar presented on July 11, 2019, https://www.youtube.com/playlist?list=PLU8c735-naXl6CvF1ESm_7Ur7c8JzWTRj.

Volek, Jeff S., Matthew J. Sharman, Dawn M. Love, Neva G. Avery, et al. "Body Composition and Hormonal Responses to a Carbohydrate-Restricted Diet." *Metabolism* 51, no. 7 (July 2002): 864–70, doi:10.1053/meta.2002.32037.

Westman, Eric C., Emily Maguire, and William S. Yancy Jr. "Ketogenic Diets as Highly Effective Treatments for Diabetes Mellitus and Obesity." Ed. Dominic P. D'Agostino. *Oxford Medicine Online* (November 2016), doi:10.1093/med/9780190497996.003.0037.

———. "Ketogenic Diets as Highly Effective Treatments for Diabetes Mellitus and Obesity." In *Ketogenic Diet and Metabolic Therapies: Expanded*

Roles in Health and Disease, ed. Susan A. Masino, 362–75. New York: Oxford University Press, 2017.

Willer, Cristen J., Ellen M. Schmidt, Sebanti Sengupta, Gina M. Peloso, et al. "Discovery and Refinement of Loci Associated with Lipid Levels." *Nature Genetics* 45, no. 11 (2013): 1274–83, https://www.ncbi.nlm.nih.gov/pmc/articles/PMC3838666/.

Würtz, Peter, Qin Wang, Pasi Soininen, Antti J. Kangas, et al. "Metabolomic Profiling of Statin Use and Genetic Inhibition of HMG-CoA Reductase." *Journal of the American College of Cardiology* 67, no. 10 (2016): 1200–1210.

Yancy, William S., Maren K. Olsen, John R. Guyton, Ronna P. Bakst, and Eric C. Westman. "A Low-Carbohydrate, Ketogenic Diet versus a Low-Fat Diet to Treat Obesity and Hyperlipidemia." *Annals of Internal Medicine* 140, no. 10 (May 18, 2004): 769–77, doi:10.7326/0003-4819-140-10-200405180-00006.

Interviews and Correspondence with the Author

Ference, Brian (June 2019)

Hu, Frank (Nov. 2018)

Mayr, Manuel (Oct. 2018)

Mozaffarian, Dariush (May 2019)

Taubes, Gary (Nov. 2018)

Notes

169 **this one conducted by Virta:** Athinarayanan et al., "Long-Term Effects."

170 **recommended revised protocol:** Goss, "Ketogenic Diet."

171 **amount of ApoB:** Eckel et al., "2013 AHA/ACC Guideline."

Chapter 38: Don't consume processed meats

Sources
Works Referenced

American Institute for Cancer Research. "FAQ: Processed Meat and Cancer." AICR eNews, August 7, 2014, https://www.aicr.org/enews/2014/08-august/faq-processed-meat-and.html.

Bellavia, Andrea, Frej Stilling, and Alicja Wolk. "High Red Meat Intake and All-Cause Cardiovascular and Cancer Mortality: Is the Risk Modified by Fruit and Vegetable Intake?" *American Journal of Clinical Nutrition* 104, no. 4 (August 24, 2016): 1137–43, doi:10.3945/ajcn.116.135335.

Demeyer, Daniel, Birgit Mertens, Stefaan De Smet, and Michèle Ulens. "Mechanisms Linking Colorectal Cancer to the Consumption of (Processed) Red Meat: A Review." *Critical Reviews in Food Science and Nutrition* 56, no. 16 (May 15, 2015): 2747–66, doi:10.1080/10408398.2013.873886.

International Agency for Research on Cancer. "IARC Monographs Evaluate Consumption of Red Meat and Processed Meat." 2015, https://www.iarc.fr/wp-content/uploads/2018/07/pr240_E.pdf.

Johnson, Bradley C., Dena Zeraatkar, Mi Ah Han, Robin W. M. Vernooij, et al. "Unprocessed Red Meat and Processed Meat Consumption: Dietary Guideline Recommendations from the Nutritional Recommendations (NutriRECS) Consortium." *Annals of Internal Medicine* (October 1, 2019), doi:10.7326/M19-1621.

Kolata, Gina. "Eat Less Red Meat, Scientists Said. Now Some Believe That Was Bad Advice." *New York Times*, September 30, 2019.

———. "That Perplexing Red Meat Controversy: 5 Things to Know." *New York Times*, September 30, 2019.

Larsson, S. C., and N. Orsini. "Red Meat and Processed Meat Consumption and All-Cause Mortality: A Meta-Analysis." *American Journal of Epidemiology* 179, no. 3 (October 22, 2013): 282–89, doi:10.1093/aje/kwt261.

Micha, Renata, Sarah K. Wallace, and Dariush Mozaffarian. "Red and Processed Meat Consumption and Risk of Incident Coronary Heart Disease, Stroke, and Diabetes: A Systematic Review and Meta-Analysis." HHS Author Manuscripts (May 17, 2010), doi:10.1161/CIRCULATIONAHA.109.924977.

———. "Red and Processed Meat Consumption and Risk of Incident Coronary Heart Disease, Stroke, and Diabetes Mellitus." *Circulation* 121, no. 21 (June 2010): 2271–83, doi:10.1161/circulationaha.109.924977.

Pan, An, Qi Sun, Adam M. Bernstein, Matthias B. Schulze, et al. "Red Meat Consumption and Risk of Type 2 Diabetes: 3 Cohorts of US Adults and an Updated Meta-Analysis." *American Journal of Clinical Nutrition* 94, no. 4 (August 10, 2011): 1088–96, doi:10.3945/ajcn.111.018978.

Song, Mingyang, Teresa T. Fung, Frank B. Hu, Walter C. Willett, et al. "Association of Animal and Plant Protein Intake with All-Cause and Cause-Specific Mortality." *JAMA Internal Medicine* 176, no. 10 (October 1, 2016): 1453–63, doi:10.1001/jamainternmed.2016.4182.

Williams, Kim Allan. "Plant Power: Whole Food Plant-Based Diets." Lecture presented at the American Heart Association Scientific Sessions, Chicago, IL, November 10–12, 2018.

World Health Organization. "About the Global Burden of Disease (GBD) Project." Health Statistics and Information Systems, https://www.who.int/healthinfo/global_burden_disease/about/en/ (accessed November 4, 2019).

———. "Q&A on the Carcinogenicity of the Consumption of Red Meat and Processed Meat." October 2015, https://www.who.int/features/qa/cancer-red-meat/en/.

———. "Q&A on the Carcinogenicity of the Consumption of Red Meat and Processed Meat." World Health Organization, October 2015, https://www.who.int/features/qa/cancer-red-meat/en/.

Zheng, Yan, Yanping Li, Ambika Satija, An Pan, et al. "Association of Changes in Red Meat Consumption with Total and Cause Specific Mortality among US Women and Men: Two Prospective Cohort Studies." *BMJ* (June 12, 2019): l2110, doi:10.1136/bmj.l2110.

Notes

173 **World Health Organization defines:** World Health Organization, "Q&A."

174 **same category as tobacco smoking:** Ibid.

174 **"about 34,000 cancer deaths":** World Health Organization, "About the Global Burden of Disease."

175 **2010 meta-analysis:** Micha et al., "Red and Processed Meat Consumption."

175 **Nurses' Health Study found:** Song et al., "Association of Animal and Plant Protein Intake."

176 **recent and highly controversial:** Johnson et al., "Unprocessed Red Meat and Processed Meat Consumption."

176 **front page:** Kolata, "That Perplexing Red Meat Controversy."

176 **reduction of one to six:** Kolata, "Eat Less Red Meat."

Chapter 39: Your diet doesn't have to be perfect

Sources
Works Referenced

Sicat, Jeffrey M. "An Obesity Medicine Approach to Managing Diabetes and Weight-Related Complications." Lecture presented at the Obesity Medicine Association, Washington, DC, September 29, 2018.

Notes

181 **the best I can do:** I would like to acknowledge Jeffrey Sicat's lecture presented at the Obesity Medicine Association in 2018 for this concept.

Epilogue:
In the Public Interest: Changing Our Food Environment

Sources
Works Referenced

Mozaffarian, Dariush, John Courtney, David A. Kessler, and Joon Yun. "Strengthening Nutrition Research: The Role of a National Institute of Nutrition." Lecture presented at Nutrition 2019, Boston, MA, June 11, 2019.

Rao, M., A. Afshin, G. Singh, D. Mozaffarian, et al. "Do Healthier Foods and Diet Patterns Cost More Than Less Healthy Options? A Systematic Review and Meta-Analysis." *BMJ Open* 2013;3:e004277, doi:10.1136/bmj open-2013-004277.

Yun, Joon, David A. Kessler, and Dan Glickman. "Opinion: We Need Better Answers on Nutrition." *New York Times*, February 28, 2019.

Acknowledgments

A legion of people have been generous with their time, ideas, and research in the course of my writing. I thank those whose names appear in the body of this book, including the endnotes, where you will find all those I interviewed and whose lectures I attended.

In addition, I am indebted to those whose names appear below. As is usual to state, and, in this case is true, any errors are mine alone.

Karyn Feiden and Richie Chevat stepped into the breach, rescuing me with their superlative writing skills. They understood what I wanted to say, and they understood the science. I couldn't have done it without them.

Thanks as well to the terrific writers Sheila Himmel, Maria Williams, Nell Casey, Thomas Dolinger, and Kristin Loberg.

HarperCollins has once again taken me seriously. For that I thank Julie Will and Karen Rinaldi. They are great supporters and editors. Thanks, too, to Kathy Robbins, my stalwart agent, and her colleague Janet Oshiro. We all, but especially I, have missed the brilliant Dick Todd on this outing. His life and death changed all of us.

Once again, my appreciation to Lynda and Stewart

Resnick and Dagmar Dolby for their financial support. My research has taken me to unlikely places, and they have made that possible.

The production of a book such as this one (a lot of science, a lot of research, and a lot of endnotes) is dependent on a sterling crew. A special shout-out to the patient and careful Tanya Boroff for work on the manuscript, transcription of interviews, and citation checking. I also appreciate the painstaking work of Richard Alwyn Fisher.

My thanks to Rebecca Raskin and Christina Gaugler.

Copy editors continually save me from myself. Thanks, Josh Karpf, Chris Jerome, Robert Land, and Melissa Lux.

In 2004, I talked about the value of whole grains at General Mills. I have served as an adviser to several food companies. I am the chair of the board at the Center for Science in the Public Interest (CSPI). In other words, I've been around. I would like to think that none of these contacts have influenced my work, but I leave it to the readers to decide.

I have benefited greatly from my discussions (often over a meal) with experts in the field of nutrition. Thank you, Mollie Van Lieu, Kate Fitzgerald, Jerry Mande, Gary Taubes, Dary Mozaffarian (who helped me focus on the role of starch), Ron Krauss, Brian Ference, Michael Pollan, Dean Ornish, and John Sievenpiper (who suggested to me the term *slow carbs*).

For their careful fact-checking I thank Jordan Balletto, Matt Mahony, Emily Loftis, Laura Zelko, Susan Weill, and Ghada Scruggs. Thanks to Kate Mertes and John

Beauregard for the index. I am an author who definitely needs proofreaders. Thank you, Chris Jerome, Roanne Goldfein, Elizabeth Macfie, Eliza Childs, Sheila Oakley, and Mary Bagg.

Jacket designer Chip Kidd always gets it. Thank you, Chip.

My appreciation for legal expertise goes to Laura Handman; for permissions editing to Sheri Gilbert; and for Library of Congress classifications, to Lisa Rowlison de Ortiz.

Thank you to Elizabeth Dupuis for access to the University of California, Berkeley Library.

My thanks to Yelena Nesbit, Tina Andreadis, and Brian Perrin for their mastery of media and marketing.

At my academic home, the University of California, San Francisco, my thanks to Changzhao Feng in accounting. And a heartfelt thank you for the support of Dean Talmadge King.

My mother, Roz, died in 2019. Now there is no one left to complain about the reviews (she even griped about the good ones) and bookstore placement. I miss her and my father. I'm glad I have my sister, Barbara, with whom to share the memories.

Love and thanks, as always, to Elise, Mike, Lena, and David; to Ben and Mollie; and to Suzanne.

And to Paulette, today, tomorrow, and forever.

Index

Index

Index

Index

About the Author

DAVID A. KESSLER, MD, served as commissioner of the U.S. Food and Drug Administration under presidents George H. W. Bush and Bill Clinton. He is a pediatrician and has been the dean of the medical schools at Yale and the University of California, San Francisco. He is a graduate of Amherst College, the University of Chicago Law School, and Harvard Medical School.

Read More by
David A. Kessler

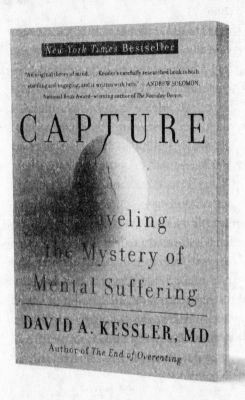

"**A breakthrough book.** In a world of increasingly specialized knowledge, it takes a particular gift and some stubbornness to cut across the fields of neuroscience, psychiatry, philosophy and psychology and to ask the fundamental question: Why it is that we can allow our best selves to be captured by and torpedoed by thoughts and actions that sink us? ... [Kessler's] ultimate answer is profound and one that could be life-changing and life-saving."

—ABRAHAM VERGHESE, MD,
author of *Cutting for Stone*

 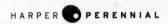